LIZ EARLE'S

QUICK GUIDES

Successful Slimming

BOXTREE

Advice to the Reader

Before following any dietary advice contained in this book, it is recommended that you consult your doctor if you suffer from any health problems or special condition or are in any doubt.

First published in Great Britain in 1994 by Boxtree Limited,
Broadwall House, 21 Broadwall, London SE1 9PL

10 9 8 7 6 5 4 3 2

ISBN: 1 85283 984 8

Text design by Blackjacks
Cover design by Hammond Hammond

Printed and Bound in Great Britain by Cox & Wyman Ltd.,
Reading, Berkshire

A CIP catalogue entry for this book is available from
the British Library

Contents

Acknowledgements

I am grateful to Sarah Hamilton-Fleming for helping to produce this book. I am also indebted to the talented team at Boxtree, Rosemary Sandberg and Claire Bowles Publicity for their unfailing enthusiasm and support.

Introduction

The last few years have seen more diet books and regimes to lose weight than on any other subject. So why the need for yet another guide? Well, if any of these books, tapes, videos or charts actually worked we'd all have reached our target weight years ago. As it is, 60 percent of all women see themselves as being overweight. I know how it feels. I was one of them. Over the years I must have tried virtually every fad diet under the sun. There was the week on eggs and grapefruit, meal replacement bars, food combining and even a stint with Weight Watchers. Sure, I lost a few pounds here and there, but after a few months they would come creeping back on.

The only answer to long-term, successful slimming is to get to grips with the causes of weight gain and to re-educate yourself with healthy eating habits. The knowledge has taken me years to acquire, but now I no longer have a problem with my weight. Nor do I count calories, worry about which foods to eat or live on starvation rations. I have simply switched to fresh, wholesome foods, choose low-fat options, try to curb a naturally sweet tooth, watch how much I drink and take a good deal more exercise. We all know these factors are important – so this *Quick Guide* is hardly revolutionary. What I hope it will do is convince you that fad diets simply don't work and that losing weight too quickly can be downright dangerous. So take the long-term view. Read the facts and decide for yourself. After all – you have nothing to lose but your excess weight. Good luck!

Liz Earle

1

Diet Damage

The slimming business is booming. In 1992, we spent more than £1.5 billion on slimming foods and products. Profits for the food industry are enormous and huge amounts of money are also spent encouraging us to buy 'slimming' aids. But liquid 'diet' drinks, meal replacement bars and small sachets of dehydrated granules are not a natural, vital way of eating. Although highly profitable, they do not teach us the simple eating habits that will result in a successful, long-term weight loss.

Ninety-five percent of us who follow a commercial dieting regime put the weight back on, and more, when we stop.

We are far more likely to lose £££s than pounds and there is slim evidence that any of the meal replacements and very low calorie regimes work in the long run.

The Health Education Authority's yearly nutrition education budget of under £1 million is dwarfed by the £600 million or more the food industry spends each year on advertising. Manufactured foods are, pound for pound, less nutritious and tend to be more fattening than their raw ingredients. They are too often high in sugar, fat, salt and too low in fibre. For example, a large portion of McDonald's Chicken McNuggets and chips has over 75g of fat, yet only 4g of fibre. One of the aims of this *Quick Guide* is to give you the information to make the informed food choices that will lead to your own permanent weight loss. It also sets out the unbiased, unequivocal facts of successful slimming. This book gives you the truth, the whole truth and nothing but the truth.

Diets Can Damage Your Health

The danger of dieting is in the fast and furious approach. It is a biological fact of life that the more quickly you lose weight, the faster you will put it back on. Slow, sustained weight loss is the *only* way to reduce body fat and not lose essential lean muscle tissue. For a diet to be truly effective, any weight loss must be slow in order to be sustained. Weight loss must also be based on the newly recognised principles of nutritious eating and should be combined with a regular exercise regime. This *Quick Guide* is not a quick fix. However, it does offer you the knowledge that will help you to achieve significant, long-term weight loss for a lifetime.

Why Most Diets Don't Work

According to the Government's 1992 *Dietary and Nutritional Survey of British Adults*, 12 percent of all women and 4 percent of all men are following a rigid dieting regime at any one moment in time. The average length of these diets is six and a half weeks for women and ten weeks for men. So why aren't all these diets working? The plain, unpalatable truth is that short-term, fad diets simply don't lead to long-term weight loss. In fact, they are quite likely to cause more harm than good. This is because short-term dieting triggers the damaging Yo-Yo effect. For example, if you start a fad diet that only allows you to eat a few hundred calories a day, the body believes it is at risk of starvation and quickly responds by conserving energy. This leads to a lowering of our basic metabolic rate, which controls how quickly we burn our food as fuel.

The problem with lowering our metabolism is that the body adapts and learns to survive on fewer calories. Scientists have now recognised that once the metabolism has been lowered by frugal eating, it is hard to boost it back to its previous level when you stop the diet. During a period of intense food restriction you might only be eating around 1,000 calories a day, so the body becomes adept at functioning on this low calorific intake. This means that when you return to your previous calorie intake of around 2,000 calories a day, the body stores the extra calories in the form of fat. Not only will your original weight loss quickly return, but you are also likely to end up feeling constantly hungry and so pile on the pounds more easily than before. This Yo-Yo rebound at the end of a period of dieting is one of the key reasons why so many diets don't work in the long term. The long-term risk factors of crash dieting followed by weight gain also dangerously increase the risk of heart disease and strokes.

In addition to messing up our metabolism and damaging our health, American researchers have found that being on a strict diet actually encourages fat cells to flourish! This is because when we severely restrict our eating, the body protects itself against possible famine by actually storing more fat. Very low calorie diets simply increase the efficiency of fat storage, so extreme restriction of eating boosts unwanted fat cells. While this does not mean that we can lose weight by living on cream cakes and chips, it does show that long-term, successful slimming requires a change in tactics from conventional calorie counting.

The slimming industry's promotion of unhealthy fad diets is quite simply morally unacceptable. The relentless promotion of so-called diet products puts many millions of women under intense pressure to conform to the advertiser's pin-thin size eight models, and to feel inadequate if they cannot attain the 'ideal' shape. There is no doubt that faddy eating habits and society's obsession with the svelte female form must also take some blame for the dramatic rise in serious eating disorders over the last decade. It is therefore important to put any kind of weight-loss regime into perspective. What we want is firm, fit, healthy bodies. Looking anorexic is not attractive.

2

Think Slim

An important part of dieting is examining our attitude to food. We should not feel guilty about what we eat or simply blame our size on all the foods which we enjoy most. If your favourite food is cheese, which has a very high fat content, then you should not feel the need to cut it out of your diet completely, merely limit the amount of cheese you eat each week. There is no point depriving yourself of all the foods you love best just because they are high in calories, as this will probably make you depressed about your diet. If you are fed up with your diet, this can provoke you into finding comfort in the very foods which you are trying to avoid eating in the first place.

Whatever diet you are on, it is very important to make sure that you are getting your daily requirements of all the vitamins and minerals. Eat plenty of fresh fruit and vegetables, which are great to snack on between meals. To feel healthy and fit everyone needs a healthy diet with all the essential nutrients including certain fats. For those who are on low fat diets, you must have some polyunsaturated fat in your diet. Some types of fat, known as essential fatty acids, are extremely good for us and we cannot function properly without them. These fats are found in vegetable oils extracted from olives, peanuts, avocados and sunflowers etc. The requirement for essential fatty acids varies with the total fat content of the diet, but they should be at least a quarter of all fats consumed. After water, which makes roughly up to 70 percent of the total weight of an adult human being, fat is the most abundant substance found in the human body.

The exact amount of fat in the body is influenced by diet, exercise, age, gender and genetic disposition and it can vary from 5 to 60 percent. Most people are made up of between 15 and 22 percent fat. Diets high in calories from any source such as refined sugars, starches, proteins or saturated fat, tend to put on extra weight and all concentrated foods increase fat deposition.

In contrast, those on diets high in fibre and leafy vegetables tend to keep slim. Several official bodies in the US recommend that our fat intake should be 30 percent of the total calories we consume daily. This 30 percent should be split equally into saturated fats, monounsaturated fats and essential fatty acids, each type of fat being 10 percent of our daily calorie intake. To really get the best from any diet, it is important to retrain the way you think about food; a cream cake or a chocolate bar should not necessarily be looked upon as a treat and your only solace, because not only are they very high in sugar and calories, they are also unhealthy. The first priority of your diet is to feel good, and this can only be achieved by eating delicious healthy foods. Remember that, whatever diet you are on, it is important to drink plenty of water, preferably mineral water.

Now let us take a look at some of the most popular diets.

3

Which Diet?

Weight Watchers

This is possibly the most popular diet in the UK, probably because it is very clearly set out and all the work is done for you. It was developed about thirty years ago in the US by Jean Nidetch and was adopted by Bernice Western in the UK twenty-six years ago. The Weight Watchers diet is designed to encourage weight loss as well as *retraining* slimmers to eat healthier food. This is basically achieved by watching the amount of food consumed each day, cutting down on meal portions, and counting each calorie. Weight Watchers provides different ideas for meal patterns and recipes and their convenience meals and ingredients can be bought in the shops. Psychological support is provided through regular group meetings with other slimmers, and there is also a magazine which offers more advice and ideas for meals. Weight Watchers covers practically every aspect of slimming, providing a safe way to lose weight, by teaching slimmers to switch to healthier foods and taking lifestyle and psychology into account.

A TYPICAL DAY'S MENU

Breakfast – 120ml orange juice, porridge made with water, 150ml skimmed milk, tea or coffee.

Lunch – poached egg with 90g grilled mushrooms, slice of toast with margarine, one pear, tea or coffee.

Dinner – grilled lamb chop served with 90g onions sautéed in 1tsp oil, 180g noodles and 90g cooked carrots, one medium orange, tea or coffee.

THE PROS

* People on the programme can attend meetings in their area and are given instructions on how to record weight, body measurements and goals as well as how to detail the different food groups and those foods to be eaten each day.
* The daily diet is explained in great detail and advice is given on how to plan celebration meals and what to eat when in a restaurant.
* Advice is given on exercise and on the psychology of slimming and how to change your self-image.
* Weekly meetings allow the slimmers to 'weigh-in' and they are rewarded and encouraged with every half stone lost. Merely having the knowledge that you have to state your weight at a one-to-one consultation with the leader is often enough motivation to lose weight. This is followed by a half-hour group discussion.
* Slimmers are given the opportunity to buy diet scales, detailed food charts and special recipe books.
* The diet is planned by nutritionists and is in line with current medical advice from the Department of Health.
* After the initial three weeks, weight loss should be at the rate of two pounds per week and if the slimmer exceeds this they are advised to consult their group leader to prevent drastic weight loss or endangering their health.
* Children between the ages of ten and sixteen who wish to follow the diet require written consent from their doctor, who must also advise them of a goal weight.

THE CONS

* Every aspect of the diet is so clearly outlined that there is a lot of literature to get through, as well as numerous charts and checklists to fill in.

* It is suggested that in the early stages of the diet each portion must be weighed, which is very time consuming.
* Those who have any prior knowledge of nutrition may find the system merely repeats what they already know.
* You will find the group sessions pointless if you do not enjoy participating as a member of a group.
* To join Weight Watchers a registration fee has to be paid. Membership lasts for ten weeks and each weekly meeting has to be paid for – even those weeks that are missed (unless a member has given prior notice of their wish to discontinue).

The F-Plan

This high-fibre diet became famous in the 1980s when it literally took Britain by storm. The two basic rules of the F-Plan diet are: reduce your calories and increase your intake of dietary fibre. There are plenty of low calorie fibre-rich meals for slimmers to choose from which are generally very filling. Fibre is found in a wide range of cereal, fruit and vegetables and a little amount of these foods can easily fill us up, and can therefore make weight loss easier. Eating foods rich in fibre speeds the excretion of waste through the bowels, thereby preventing constipation and certain diseases associated with the bowel. High-fibre foods can also lead to weight loss because they are not as fully digested as other foods. It is claimed that this leads to fewer calories being utilised by the body, which then has to turn to its own stores of surplus fat to get the energy it needs.

A TYPICAL DAY'S MENU

Breakfast – a bowl of bran cereal with a small sliced banana and semi-skimmed milk.

Lunch – vegetable and lentil soup with a wholemeal roll. If you crave something sweet, dried apricots are very high in fibre and have a sweet taste.
Dinner – lamb chop with new potatoes, butter beans and tomatoes.

THE PROS

* High-fibre foods cleanse your internal system and prevent constipation by speeding up the waste-removal process.
* It differs from other diets in the way that the foods are very filling and do not leave you with that half-empty feeling.
* The combination of unrefined carbohydrate, vegetables and fruit is just what many nutritionists recommend we should all eat.
* It is an inexpensive, convenient and flexible eating regime.

THE CONS

* The high levels of fibre may cause uncomfortable bloating or wind in people who are not used to eating so much fibre.
* Eating fibre in the form of bran can reduce the body's ability to absorb useful minerals eaten shortly before or afterwards, although the level of bran in wholemeal bread does not have a significant effect in this respect.
* It is not simply a matter of eating any foods which are high in fibre, as some of these are also high in calories, for example dried apricots, avocados and nuts are all good sources of fibre but they are also fairly high in calories. So if you want to lose weight significantly every calorie has to be counted.
* The original F-Plan diet is now very dated as it was written in the early 1980s. The emphasis is definitely

more on weight loss than health and the recommended foods and recipes are full of processed foods, although there are plenty of natural sources of fibre.

Food Combining

This type of diet was invented by an American doctor more than seventy years ago, and it is presently enjoying a revival. This diet is not designed solely for those who want to lose weight, but it is a good general eating plan. It is not a fast-acting 'fad' diet, as it is designed to shift weight steadily. Doctor Hay, who invented the diet, believed that starch and protein are treated differently by the digestive system, and so should, therefore, never be eaten together in the same meal. This of course means that many traditional dishes are immediately ruled out of the diet, such as roast dinners with meat and potatoes, spaghetti bolognese and most sandwiches. Grains such as rice, pasta and bread as well as potatoes can be eaten with vegetables, but not with meat, fish or dairy products which are all high in protein. These protein foods can in turn be eaten with vegetables but not with foods containing a lot starch. This diet may mean re-thinking all your meals, but many of those who have tried it claim that the system enables you to control weight effortlessly.

A TYPICAL DAY'S DIET

Breakfast – home-made muesli containing oatmeal, grated almonds and brazil nuts, raisins, linseed, pumpkin and sunflower seeds, all soaked in apple juice and lemon juice, with a grated apple added just before serving.
Lunch – salad with avocado dip.
Dinner – a protein meal of grilled fish with a large green vegetable and herb salad, with yoghurt or olive oil dressing.

The pros

* Food combining puts a lot of emphasis on eating vegetables, fruit and unrefined carbohydrates, coupled with a moderate fat intake, which amounts to extremely healthy eating.
* The meals do not require a great deal of cooking because most of the ingredients used are fresh.
* The idea of only combining certain food types is a simple one to grasp and there is no need to weigh every portion and count every calorie because the foods recommended in the diet have low fat and sugar contents.
* Food combining is a long-term eating plan rather than a 'fad' diet and is more likely than many other diets to lead to permanent weight loss and a healthy body provided it is stuck to.

The cons

* Almost every eating habit has to be changed; no more cheese or ham sandwiches, no meat with potatoes and no pasta or rice with fish or meat.
* Eating out can be a problem because this diet rejects many traditional recipes, but it is by no means impossible.
* There is no scientific basis as yet to confirm that food combining really does work, but many of those who have tried it are convinced it does.

Hip and Thigh Diet

If you ask most women which part of their body needs to lose weight the most, even the slimmest woman would probably say her thighs. The area around the hips and thighs is always the most difficult place to shift fat from and the hip and thigh diet targets this area through a combination of a very low fat diet and exercise. Research has shown that female fat cells are larger than their male counterparts, and have greater fat-storing abilities. Women are also prone to fat because they are influenced by oestrogen which feeds the fat cells of the hips and thighs. Therefore, to stop fat being stored in this way, the obvious thing to do is to eat less fat. The aim behind this diet is to cut out virtually all fat from the diet and retrain the slimmer to eat healthier foods. The diet is not drastically low in calories and so it is suitable for a long-term eating regime. It is based on three meals a day with one three-course meal which should keep any hunger pangs at bay. This should not cause any change in your metabolic rate which often decreases in those eating very little each day, thus causing a Yo-Yo effect.

A TYPICAL DAY'S MENU

Breakfast – 20g (3/4oz) All-Bran, one small sliced banana, and skimmed milk from a daily allowance of 280ml (half a pint).
Lunch – jacket potato with 225g (8oz) tin of baked beans.
Dinner – leek and potato soup, chicken curry with brown rice, meringue basket with raspberries and low fat raspberry yoghurt or low fat fromage frais.

THE PROS

* Eating less saturated fat is a vital part of keeping healthy as it reduces the risk of heart disease and other degenerative diseases.
* There is no time-consuming calorie counting involved.
* A low fat diet is not difficult to achieve if dairy products are avoided, and there are countless quick and easy low fat meals to make.
* You can even enjoy a sensible amount of alcohol on this type of diet.
* Unlimited amounts of vegetables can be eaten.

The cons

* Long-term low fat diets can cause deficiencies in certain essential fatty acids found in vegetable oils which can result in countless different problems, from PMT to dry skin. All oils, butters, margarines and most nuts are forbidden, so to maintain optimum nutrition those who are on this type of low fat diet should take a capsule of evening primrose oil and fish oil daily, which only amounts to five calories.
* Low fat diets are unlikely to provide the required amounts of vitamins and minerals, especially if you are pregnant, and so it is best to take a multi-vitamin pill as a safeguard.
* The diet focuses on weight loss rather than on learning how to improve your health through eating more nutritious foods. As an example, it does not rule out eating certain desserts which have a high sugar content.
* Low fat dairy produce can be boring and taste bland. All dairy produce should also be avoided by those with a milk intolerance.

The Scarsdale Diet

This is a fourteen-day diet with a specific menu for each day and it is suggested that you spend two weeks on the diet followed by two weeks off. The theory behind the diet is that, in the absence of carbohydrate, you can eat large amounts of meat, fish, cheese or eggs without the calories being made available to the body in a suitable form for storing fat. The vegetables permitted are all very low in carbohydrates but are high in vitamins, minerals and fibre. The eating plan is completely inflexible and you must stick exactly to each day's menu.

A TYPICAL DAY'S MENU

Breakfast – half a grapefruit and one slice of wholemeal toast and black coffee or tea.

Lunch – as much low fat cottage cheese as you want, courgettes or string beans and two eggs which have been cooked without fat, and one slice of wholemeal toast, with black coffee or tea.

Dinner – as much grilled or roasted skinless chicken as you want with spinach, green peppers and beans, and coffee or tea.

THE PROS

* Weight loss is quick and it is therefore a good way to kick-start a general change for the better in eating habits.
* You will not feel hungry because of the unlimited amounts of high protein foods allowed.
* Not much cooking is involved except for grilling or roasting meat.

THE CONS

* The regime is completely inflexible and each day's diet must be adhered to. This makes eating out a problem.
* A lot of the initial weight loss is due to liquid loss and will be replaced as soon as the slimmer moves to the lower protein regime.
* The diet is extremely low in cereal fibre and carbohydrate. Experts now recommend that 50 percent of our daily calorie intake should come from carbohydrates and only 15 percent from protein. This diet is, therefore, unhealthy in the long term.
* It is totally unsuitable for vegetarians.

Meal Replacements

These involve eating ready-made nutritious drinks and snacks instead of proper meals. This way the overall calorie intake is reduced dramatically to around 1,000 calories a day. Some companies offer these food replacements as an alternative to breakfast and lunch and then you cook your own evening meal. This type of diet controls exactly what you eat so there is no guesswork involved. The worry with this is that the meal replacements are no substitute for real food and do not contain the essential nutrients we all need. However, many of these products do contain a good amount of additional nutrients to make up for this.

A TYPICAL DAY'S MENU

Breakfast – a 'nutritious' milk drink.
Lunch – a 'nutritious' soup.
Dinner – turkey and broccoli followed by a grapefruit.

THE PROS

* Good meal replacement products stress on their labels that they should not be a slimmer's sole source of nutrition.
* These ready-prepared meal substitutes and snacks make life very simple as there is no calorie counting or special recipe following involved. It is best suited for those who lead busy lives and do not have the time or the energy to follow a more complex form of diet.
* Buying these food replacements may actually save you money as the meal replacements are generally cheap and you only have to shop for one meal's food for each day.
* Many of the products available are fortified with vitamins and minerals and some even contain the recommended daily requirements of these.

THE CONS

* Because meal replacements contain so few calories, weight drops off at an accelerated rate. This can cause serious health problems.
* This regime, like so many others, is so strict as to cause problems when eating out.
* As soon as you have lost the weight that you wanted to lose, and resume a normal diet, then the chances are that you will put the weight straight back on.
* These meal replacements offer no advice about maintaining your new weight while eating properly.
* Many of the low calorie nutrition bars available contain a high amount of sugar which will satisfy cravings for sweet food, but it would be much healthier to snack on a piece of fruit instead.
* Going straight from eating three meals a day to eating only one and meal replacements can seriously disrupt your digestive system. It is best to cut down on meals gradually, perhaps by reducing the portion sizes, and then introduce the meal replacements at the same pace.
* Reducing calorie intake to 1,000 calories a day is known to cause the metabolism to slow down, which is counterproductive. Once the metabolism has slowed down, the calories do not get burned off at a good rate and are, therefore, stored as fat.
* Meal replacements do not encourage you to shop for healthy, low fat alternatives or encourage using healthier cooking techniques for the future.

The Detox Diet

This is a very short-term diet for those who want to rid their body of toxins, perhaps after a particularly heavy consumption of alcohol and food.

Detox diets can benefit us all, whether we need to lose weight or not. The environment of the modern Western world is a constant source of toxins not only through the heavily processed foods that we consume, but also through the increasingly polluted atmosphere. Most fruit and vegetables we eat are sprayed with pesticides, so even those on very healthy diets cannot escape toxins altogether. The only way to ensure that we do not consume them through our food is to buy organically grown products. A detox diet usually involves eating one kind of fruit and drinking lots of mineral water which is the best way to flush out the system, ridding the body of all toxins. Another method of detoxing the body is through a method known as juicing, which involves drinking the freshly made juice from a particular fruit or vegetable and nothing else. Some of those who promote this type of diet also claim that the enzymes in particular fruit can actually improve weight loss.

A TYPICAL DAY'S MENU

Breakfast – an apple and a glass of mineral water.
Lunch – two bananas and a couple of glasses of mineral water.
Dinner – a fruit salad made from pineapple and strawberries.

THE PROS

* Detox diets give your body a well-earned break from toxins, giving your internal system a complete spring clean which no other type of diet can do.
* Detox diets may kick-start your body into eliminating cellulite which is caused by the build-up of toxins in the body.

* The diet only lasts for a couple of days leaving you feeling fresh and revived.
* It is very cheap and simple to follow and there is absolutely no cooking involved.
* This diet will certainly solve any constipation problems.
* Fresh fruit is an excellent source of many vitamins and minerals.

THE CONS

* It is not a long-term slimming diet and is really only designed to rid the body of toxins temporarily. To maintain excellent health, the detox diet must be repeated every few months.
* Detoxing is not a method suited to those who lead busy lives and who, therefore, need as much energy as they can muster.
* You will probably experience headaches, which is a sign that the body is eliminating toxins, in the same way that you suffer from a headache if you have a hangover.
* While detoxing you won't have much energy to go out and do things, so it is best to rest at home while your body goes through this process.
* This diet must not be continued for more than a few days because the body is not getting all the nutrients it needs to function properly.

The Mediterranean Diet

The people of the Mediterranean have really got the right idea when it comes to what we should be eating. They have one of the lowest rates of heart disease in the world and yet they eat moderate amounts of cheese, meat and red wine. The key to their good health lies in the olive oil which is used in liberal amounts in their cooking. Mediterranean people also eat a lot of fresh fish and other fresh produce, and a lot less processed food. Recent research has shown that vegetable oils such as olive oil and fish oils contain essential fatty acids which are needed by the body to produce prostaglandins. These are hormone-like chemicals which are responsible for regulating cellular activity and, thereby, preventing heart attacks and strokes and many other conditions. Small amounts of alcohol have also been shown to produce prostaglandins in the body. The Mediterranean diet is not a diet in the weight-loss sense of the word and its eating plans are not rigid. Instead, it offers the freedom to choose from healthy foods while leaving out the saturated fats, sugars and processed foods of which the average diet is full.

A typical day's menu

Breakfast – a selection of fruit and perhaps some fresh bread with some fruit juice or water.

Lunch – salad niçoise with tuna, anchovies and olives and an olive oil dressing with a couple of glasses of water to drink.

Dinner – large green or red pepper stuffed with rice, minced meat, tomato and herbs, all soaked in olive oil (before baking) and served with salad and some fresh bread. A glass of red wine can be drunk with the meal.

The pros

* This diet has endless varieties of healthy meals to choose from and it is certainly not boring.
* There are many healthy Mediterranean dishes on offer in countless restaurants so eating out should not interfere with the diet.
* The Mediterranean diet is designed more for good health than for weight loss and this should always be the order of priority.

* Most Mediterranean meals are easy to make as lots of the foods used are eaten fresh; pasta dishes especially are extremely quick and easy to prepare.
* The health benefits of this diet are overwhelming, and not just in lowering cholesterol and blood pressure, many who have tried it claim that it helped relieve their arthritic pain. This is probably due to the high content of essential fatty acids in the form of vegetable and fish oils.
* Although the diet will not encourage great weight loss, the change in eating habits which it promotes should help to keep the pounds off permanently.

THE CONS

* Those with serious weight problems will probably need a more rigid diet to follow which provides calorie guidelines.
* If you are expecting quick weight loss then you will be disappointed.
* The basics of the Mediterranean diet should really be incorporated into your daily eating plans permanently. This means cutting out processed foods, fast food and all stodgy British meals. But this con is really a pro in terms of long-term good health.

The Stone Age Diet

This diet undermines the very premise on which practically every other diet exists, namely that calorie counting works. The idea behind this primitive diet is that starving yourself of calories is no key to losing weight permanently. The diet involves eating more natural, organically grown foods and less fat and sugar. Almost all manufactured foods should be avoided as, after being processed, many foods lose some or even all of their natural nutrients. Many food manufacturers claim that their products are nutritious, but they have merely added synthetically produced vitamins and minerals to their products which are no replacement for the real thing. The diet also excludes all refined and processed oils as well as refined sugar and simple carbohydrates such as white bread and most packaged cereals. It consists of eating high-fibre foods and is really a 1990s version of the F-Plan diet, except that the emphasis is more on health than calorie counting. The foods recommended are whole fruits, vegetables, whole grains, green leafy vegetables, beans, herbs and root vegetables. This eating regime is designed to enable you to shed excess fat without making you drastically thinner and lacking in energy.

A TYPICAL DAY'S MENU

Breakfast – raisin and oatmeal porridge made with water and concentrated apple juice.
Lunch – thick vegetable soup and a wholemeal roll.
Dinner – vegetable curry made with potatoes, pumpkin and carrots and served with wholemeal rice.

THE PROS

- This diet does not encourage depriving your body of the energy foods which it requires as most diets do.
- Consuming large amounts of protein and low amounts of fat and sugar is in line with current nutritional guidelines.
- There is no time-consuming calorie counting involved.
- The diet is fairly flexible.
- An excellent long-term health and weight-loss regime.

THE CONS

- Because processed foods are not allowed in the diet, it means buying almost everything fresh and then cooking it which can be time consuming, and involves careful and frequent shopping.

* You need to shake off the habits of a lifetime and be prepared to try a wealth of new foods like tofu, beansprouts, pulses and grains.
* The diet also encourages the slimmer to reverse 'normal' eating habits by having large breakfasts and small dinners (these last two cons are really pros in the long run).

4

Low Fat, High Vitality

The most successful diet of all is based on the simple low fat, high-vitality principle, and I believe it to be the best option. It is entirely safe for every member of the family to follow. This is because it is based on sound nutritional know-how and well-balanced eating. Whether you would like to lose four pounds or forty pounds, the principle ensures that the fat not only falls off, but that it stays off forever. Low fat recipes can be found in every modern, healthy eating recipe book and are easy for anyone to follow. They can be adapted to suit teenagers, working women, business dinners, eating out, entertaining, late-night snackers, invalids and the elderly. What is more, once you have achieved your target weight, you simply need to stick to the few golden rules of healthy eating to ensure that those excess pounds never return.

The principles of any successful slimming regime are remarkably simple: eat less and do more! But within this obvious statement there are many factors that can work to make our lives and weight loss easier.

The Fat Factor

Of all the foods we should be most aware of, fat is the number one enemy of the lean body. Fat contains the highest number of calories at 9 kcals per gram than any other type of food. This compares to protein (4 kcals per gram) and carbohydrate (3.75 kcals per gram). This means that it only takes a few grams of fat to start clocking up the calories. By contrast, we can eat almost three times as much carbohydrate as fat – and still lose weight! This is one reason why you will never feel hungry while following this carbohydrate-rich eating regime. Although calorie counting has its critics because it does not take into account the type of food and how it is used in the body (for example, carbohydrates tend to be used as fuel, whereas fats are quickly stored), many of us are happy with the habit of counting calories. Personally, I prefer not to have to approach each meal with a calculator before eating, although I will concede that calorie counting is a useful tool for getting to grips with the nutritional value of different foods.

The average adult on any weight-loss regime should aim for an intake of 1,500-2,000 calories a day, depending on frame size, sex and daily energy expenditure. Bear in mind that when a recipe states that it contains a certain number of 'calories' it actually means kilocalories (a kilocalorie is 1,000 calories). So, if a dish has 200 kilocalories it is actually 200,000 calories!

How to Reach Your Weight Goal

Most of us don't need weight-loss charts to tell us that we need to lose a few pounds, or more. The testing time for our own personal body shape comes when we are in the changing room trying to squeeze into a new size twelve outfit, when buttons on a jacket begin to bulge or when a zip breaks under the strain of our great girth. We all know just by looking in the mirror that we need to lose weight. Unfortunately, research carried out by the National Toxicology Centre in Arkansas, USA, suggests that being *slightly underweight* is actually better for the body. This is because the system has to work less hard to digest food and eliminate toxic and excess materials. Over-eating, bingeing and sheer greed all place a strain on our body, so being a few pounds under our target weight should not be seen as a major problem.

However, one of the first rules of this *Quick Guide* is to stop weighing yourself more than once a fortnight. It is much more important to lose inches by firming up the body with exercise than it is to lose a few pounds of retained water. Lean muscle weighs *more* than fat and given the choice, I would far rather be fitter and leaner but weigh more than a less fit, plumper person who might actually weigh less than me. It is how you look and feel that is important, not what the scales say. Having said that, it is useful to have some kind of rough guidelines to follow regarding weight. The chart below will give you an indication of the optimum weight for your height. However, bear in mind that it is only an indication.

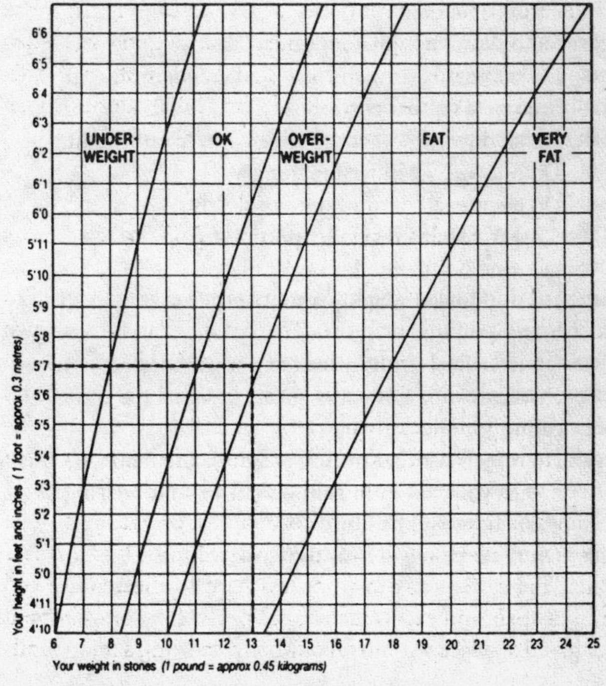

Successful Slimming Golden Rules

Before you start your new healthier eating regime:

Do's

* Do believe that this time, your diet will work for you
* Do take one day at a time
* Do forget the 'starvation' idea and work towards vitality eating
* Do look forward to slow, permanent weight loss
* Do develop a life-long love of fruits and vegetables
* Do ditch the scales
* Do set realistic goals and reward your own efforts with a food-free treat
* Do be patient with your body
* Do make friends with your local greengrocer and become a regular customer
* Do sit down to eat at the table – never eat standing up
* Do only eat when feeling hungry
* Do chew each mouthful more slowly
* Do serve yourself smaller portions
* Do leave a little food on your plate
* Do use smaller plates – a simple trick that fools the brain
* Do have fresh fruit instead of a sugary dessert
* Do clean your teeth after meals to signal the end of eating
* Do remember that muscle weighs more than fat – this means you may even gain weight while exercising but your shape will be leaner
* Do think positive! This time you will succeed.

Don'ts

* Don't panic! Successful slimming takes time and is not about major food deprivation
* Don't skip meals, your body needs a constant energy supply
* Don't feed your fat cells with more fat
* Don't expect results overnight – the more slowly you lose weight, the longer you will keep it off
* Don't eat late, your body will not be able to burn up the calories before bedtime
* Don't weigh yourself more than once a fortnight
* Don't eat sweets or chocolate as a pick-me-up
* Don't wear elasticated waistbands – they encourage you to over-eat!
* Don't read or watch TV while eating
* Don't drink with meals. Drink liquids half an hour before or after eating
* Don't ever have seconds
* Don't visit the supermarket more than once a week – menu planning in advance means you are less likely to buy extra treats
* Don't ever feel guilty about eating – your body needs food, but it needs the *right* kinds of food

5

The Fat Factor

A low fat diet is the number one improvement you will make to achieve weight loss for life and encourage lasting good health. Fats are the cause of excess body fat – not too much starch or carbohydrates. A minimum fat intake is a fundamental part of healthy eating and is even more of a priority than the other diet issues of sugar, fibre, salt and cholesterol intake. That is not to say that these are not important, just that they are secondary to the fundamental habit of eating much less fat. Remember – fat cells love fat – so don't feed it to them!

High Fat Foods vs Low Fat Foods

High Fat Foods	Low Fat Foods
Cream	Pasta
Butter	Beans and pulses
Cheese	Fish and seafood
Red meat	Breakfast cereals
Egg yolks	Bread
Full-fat milk	Fruit and vegetables

Fat Types

All fats are made up of fatty acids and contain exactly the same number of calories. Fats and oils are equally fattening. However, some fat is far worse for building a healthy body than others. Understanding the vital differences between our everyday fats and oils makes it easy to make the changes that will lead to a leaner, healthier body. Here is the low-down on the different types of fat that we eat.

SATURATES

The reason why a fat becomes 'saturated' has to do with its chemical composition and whether there is room on the fat molecule for hydrogen to bond onto it. Saturated fats are 'fully saturated' and have no room left for extra hydrogen to climb on board. Saturated fats are more easily recognised by being mostly solid at room temperature. Animal fats, such as butter, cheese, lard, dripping, suet and the white fat on meat (including chicken skin) are all very high in saturates. Tropical vegetable oils, such as palm kernel, palm and coconut oils are also high in saturated fats (watch out for these on the ingredient labels of biscuits, cakes and peanut butter).

Conclusion: Saturated fat is the most damaging to our health and has been clearly linked to cancer and heart disease.

POLYUNSATURATES

The polyunsaturates are literally 'very-unsaturated' which means that there is plenty of room on their molecule for extra hydrogen bonds. Polyunsaturates are usually found in the form of vegetable oils. The richest sources of polyunsaturates are sunflower oil, safflower oil, corn oil and soya oil. These types of fats are thought to be less damaging to our health and they do not clog the arteries in the same way that saturated fats do. However, polyunsaturates are easily broken down by cooking and can turn into potentially dangerous peroxides, which may cause other health problems.

Recent government guidelines not only recommend that we should cut back on overall fat intake, but also suggest that a diet high in polyunsaturates may not be all that good for us. The government committee's report suggests that no more than 10 percent of our daily calories should come from polyunsaturates. It is possible to exceed this if you use sunflower spread on four slices of bread a day and also use polyunsaturated oils for frying and salad dressings. Eating plenty of vitamin E at the same time as using polyunsaturated oils is essential for good health as the vitamin E protects against the damage caused by free radicals and peroxides.

Conclusion: Small amounts of polyunsaturates are useful in the diet, but should be eaten sparingly. The more polyunsaturates we eat, the more vitamin E we need.

MONOUNSATURATES

The monounsaturate molecules have room for just one hydrogen atom to bond onto each one. These fats are probably the healthiest of all as they do not clog the arteries in the same way that saturates can. They are also more stable during frying than the polyunsaturates, so are the best for cooking with. Monounsaturates are mostly liquid at room temperatures, but may solidify if stored in the fridge (olive oil is a good example of this). Several vegetable oils are high in monounsaturates including olive, rapeseed, groundnut (peanut), hazelnut, sesame and some blended vegetable oils.

Conclusion: Probably the best of all the fats, monounsaturates can be found in many healthy foods such as avocados, oats, nuts and seeds. One of the best all-rounders for cooking is cold-pressed olive oil, which also has a healthy amount of vitamin E.

Most solid cooking fats and oils are also 100 percent fat. Fat may be 'hidden' on the label in various guises. The following are all types of fat which you should watch out for:

- partially hydrogenated oils
- vegetable oils
- palm oil
- shortening

* lard
* animal fat
* butter
* cream

Slimmers should use all fats with caution and choose soft low fat and diet spreads which are whipped with water and contain around 80 percent fat, so have slightly fewer calories. Unhydrogenated diet spreads are hard to find but can be tracked down in the better health food shops.

Fat Grams

A healthy diet should contain no more than 35 percent fat, but a weight-loss diet should contain between 20 and 25 percent fat. This level will result in long-term weight loss as well as dramatically reduce our risk of cancer and heart disease. One of the easiest ways to monitor the amount of fat we eat each day is to keep track of our fat grams. This method of weight watching is especially popular in America, where it has largely replaced calorie counting. In the United States, most foods and many restaurant menus now list their fat-gram content.

The average healthy diet consists of around 80 grams of fat a day, but this should be reduced to 20–40 grams of fat a day for dieters. Learning the fat-gram content of foods is actually more effective than counting calories, as it highlights the most fattening forms of foods. Read the labels and look out for fat grams. You can also work out the fat content of foods where it is not shown by multiplying the number of grams of fat in a portion by nine to find out how many calories of fat a serving contains.

Fat-gram Finder

HIGH FAT *Type*	*Fat grams/portion*	**LOW FAT** *Type*	*Fat grams/portion*
Pork pie	30g		
Samosa	26g		
Streaky bacon, fried	25g	Streaky bacon, grilled	20g
Steak and kidney pie	24g		
Sausages	21g	Fat-reduced sausages	11g
Pork chop, grilled	20g		
Small beefburger	20g		
Cheddar cheese	19g	Cottage cheese	2g
Thin-cut chips	17g	Thick-cut chips	8g
Small bar of chocolate	15g		
Minced beef	14g	Minced beef, fat poured off	6g
Edam cheese	13g		
Double cream	13g	Single cream	6g
Small bag of peanuts	12g		
Roast chicken, with skin	12g	Roast chicken, without skin	4g
Fish fingers, fried	11g	Fish fingers, grilled	6g
Halva	11g		
Small bag of crisps	11g	Fat-reduced crisps	7g
Butter or margarine	8g		
Roast potatoes	8g	Boiled or baked potatoes	0g

Milk:

* Full-fat milk contains 22g per pint
* Semi-skimmed milk contains 11g per pint
* Skimmed milk contains just 1g fat per pint

By contrast to many of these high fat foods, see how easy it is to trim fat grams by switching to lower fat alternatives or by changing the way we cook our food. Simple changes will dramatically alter our food's fat content.

High fat Type of food	% fat	**Low fat** Type of food	% fat
Fried courgette	90	Steamed courgette	0
Breaded and fried cod	62	Grilled cod	7
Baked potato and sour cream	60	Plain baked potato	0
Boiled potatoes and butter	53	Plain boiled potato	0
Chicken roll with mayonnaise	47	Plain chicken roll	16

Ways to cut back on fat

- Switch to skimmed or semi-skimmed milk
- Use a non-stick frying pan
- Use a squirt of sprayed oil for frying
- Cook with vegetable stock instead of shallow frying in butter
- Always trim all the visible fat from meat
- Eat more fish and poultry
- Choose lower fat cheeses, such as cottage cheese
- Use low fat yoghurt instead of evaporated milk or cream
- Steam, grill or bake whenever possible

6

Sugar Sense

We are a nation of sugarholics. Confectionery sales totalling £2,332 million in 1984 were greater than the combined sum spent on bread and cereals – and the body has no need to eat any type of sugar at all! Both brown and white sugar supply only empty calories and absolutely no nourishment whatsoever. All types of sugar are also very high in calories and, after fat, are the next most powerful diet disruptors. In addition to piling on the pounds, sugar has been linked to lowered immunity, diabetes and skin disorders. As with fat, there are many different ways to describe sugar on the labels. Some may believe that one type of sugar may be better for us than others, but the fact is that sugar, sucrose, glucose, dextrose and all the other 'oses' have no nutritional value other than feeding the body with empty worthless calories.

SUCROSE

This is the white or brown sugar used in sweets, biscuits and cakes. Sucrose comes from sugar beet and sugar cane and is itself made up of two simpler sugars called fructose and glucose.

FRUCTOSE

This is found in sugar and honey and is the sweetest tasting sugar. Fructose tastes one-third sweeter than sucrose. Buying packets of refined fructose to use instead of refined sugar (sucrose) can save a third of our sugar calories as you will need to use less of it.

GLUCOSE

This is found naturally in some foods and is also known as dextrose. Glucose gives us energy but this doesn't mean that we need sweets or sports drinks with added glucose. Our energy supplies come from complex carbohydrates, or starches, which the body breaks down into simple sugars. These are then digested and absorbed as energy. As long as we get our glucose this way we do not need to eat any type of sugar at all.

LACTOSE

This is the main sugar found in milk and other dairy products and is about one-third as sweet as sucrose.

MALTOSE

This sugar is manufactured from starch. As with all other sugars, the body eventually breaks it down into glucose.

None of the sugars has any place in a healthy eating or permanent weight loss for life regime. Not only are sugars high in calories, but they are also low in important nutrients and do not contain any vitality-giving vitamins. In terms of our health, the most important difference between the different types of sugars are those that are locked into the structure of a food (intrinsic sugars) and those that are added (extrinsic sugars). The intrinsic sugars can be found in the fruits and vegetables that also contain useful vitamins. These intrinsic sugars are not harmful to our health. Extrinsic sugars are made by processing foods to release the sugars. For example, an apple contains intrinsic sugars, but turning it into processed apple purée frees the sugars and makes them extrinsic. These 'free' sugars should be used with caution. The exception is thought to be lactose, which although it is an extrinsic sugar, is not thought to damage our health. Nutritionists talk in terms of non-milk extrinsic sugars (NME) as being the type of sugars we should especially cut down on. Remember – NME is the 'enemy' and includes all added sugars, table sugar, concentrated fruit juices and honey.

Eating a sugary snack which is 100 percent sugar means that in ten to fifteen minutes the blood sugar level dramatically rises. This initial spurt of energy is quickly followed by a more lasting low. This is because insulin is secreted when blood sugar levels are high and this stores sugar from the bloodstream in our cells. So blood sugar levels drop and leave us feeling hungrier than before. This is not a true hunger, as we only ate the sweets initially as a quick snack, but it fools the brain into believing that the stomach is empty. Sugar not only rots the teeth but can also trigger the appetite. If you have a sweet tooth and want to eat sugar, only eat it with a meal so that the rate of absorption is slowed down. Artificial sweeteners may also stimulate the appetite by triggering the release of gastric juices in the stomach in the anticipation of a raised blood glucose level. Hunger pangs may then follow as the sweeteners fail to provide any of the expected calories. For this reason it is also best to eat chemical sweeteners only at meal times.

Better still, follow these pointers to reduce sugar cravings:

* Gradually cut down the amount of sugar you use in drinks and sprinkle on cereals until you stop altogether
* Always keep a supply of fruit nearby to snack on. Seedless white grapes are the sweetest fruits and will satisfy the worst sugar cravings
* A daily supplement of the mineral dolomite may help reduce sugar cravings
* Buy reduced or no-sugar versions of foods and drinks
* Sweet brown rice (from health shops) is naturally rich in intrinsic sugars and makes a great rice pudding
* Dried fruits are high in calories because they contain concentrated fruit sugars, but a handful of raisins is better for you than a sugary snack

* Carrots are also rich in natural sugars, so keep carrot sticks in the fridge for when you feel like snacking
* When cooking, cut the amount of sugar in a recipe by at least half. You will never need as much as recipes quote
* Never ever give sugary foods or drinks to babies
* Beware of ingredients ending in 'ose' such as sucrose, dextrose etc, and of any syrups such as corn syrup

Although the amount of packet sugar we buy has almost halved in the last decade, we are still eating more of the white stuff. This is due to the switch from home baking to convenience foods and confectionery. Most of the sugars we now eat come from processed foods and drinks, such as sweetened fruit juices and cans of fizzy drinks. When buying foods that contain sugars, always check the labels first. Ingredients must by law be listed in order, with the greatest first. But by dividing sugar into many different types, such as dextrose, maltose and glucose, the individual sugars will appear lower down the list. When added together, you may find that sugar is actually the main ingredient. Foods with 'no-added sugar' or 'unsweetened' are not necessarily low in sugar. They could be foods that are naturally high in sugar or may be sweetened with concentrated fruit juices (extrinsic sugars). Food labels are often a complicated maze of weasel words and misinformation. Check out the labels in your shopping trolley and see how many actually contain sugar as the main ingredient.

Teaspoons of Sugar

Aim for less than six teaspoons of NME sugars a day – remember the body does not actually need any at all.
1 level teaspoon = 5g sugar, 1 sugar lump = 2.5g

Food	Quantity	Teaspoons
Mars bar	regular size (65g)	8.5
Coca Cola	1 can (330ml)	7.0
Danish pastry	1 (110g)	6.5
Lucozade	small bottle (250ml)	4.5
Sugar Puffs	1 bowl (40g)	4.0
Unsweetened orange juice	1 carton (200ml)	3.5
Baked beans	small tin (205g)	2.5
Tinned spaghetti	small tin (215g)	2.0

Artificial Sweeteners

As adding refined sugar to foods is to be avoided, are artificial sweeteners the answer? The answer has to be no. It is far better to retrain your taste buds to accept fewer sweet foods than become dependent on a packet of chemicals.

Britons spend around £50 million a year on artificial sweeteners, so sugar substitutes are clearly big business. Although they provide all the sweetness of sugar with none of the calories, there is a sour note about their safety. While most scientific studies have passed artificial sweeteners for safety, many critics believe that there is still cause for concern. For example, some studies show that saccharin may increase the risk of cancer and cyclamates have been banned from most European countries. In America, foods containing saccharin even carry a printed warning that it may be 'hazardous to your health'. The use of artificial sweeteners in processed foods has been growing at an alarming rate in recent years. Four out of five children have saccharin at least once a week, usually in the form of soft drinks and squashes. The UK allows manufacturers to add artificial sweeteners to foods and drinks together with refined sugar. This means that you or your child could be eating large amounts of these chemicals even if there is no 'diet' label on the product.

So what really goes into these handy-sized boxes of small white pills or useful jars of sprinkle-on sweetness? Artificial sweeteners are essentially a cocktail of chemicals. The formula on a typical well-known brand reads like the contents of a chemistry set: sodium bicarbonate, trisodium citrate, saccharin, sodium carbonate, glycine and monosodium glutamate. No wonder they don't label the ingredients on the packet – it isn't big enough!

Most artificial sweeteners are known in the food industry as *intense sweeteners.* This group contains the chemicals aspartame, acesulfame-K, cyclamates, thaumatin and saccharin. All of these are classified as food additives. The food industry may also use another group called *bulk sweeteners*, which include sorbitol, mannitol, lacitol, xylitol and isomalt. These are actually 'sweet' alcohols or polyols and occur naturally in fruit. These bulk sweeteners are also commercially produced by combining sugars such as glucose and lactose with hydrogen to harden them (in a similar way to hydrogenated fats). Their only real advantage over ordinary sugar is that they won't contribute to tooth decay, although they do contain just as many calories.

I'm afraid there is no alternative but to wean yourself off sugar and its substitutes as much as possible. You don't have to cut all sugar out of your life overnight, but start reducing the amount you eat now – grain by grain, if necessary.

7

Full of Fibre

Eating plenty of fibre-rich carbohydrates is the basis for any successful slimming regime. Carbohydrates are 'good guys' because the body stores any extra carbohydrate we eat in the form of glycogen. The body cannot make much glycogen from fatty foods. This means that the body resists making extra fat from carbohydrates until its glycogen stores are replenished. It is very hard for the body to turn carbohydrates into fat. Regular exercise means that an extra helping of pasta is unlikely to end up as fat layers on our hips and thighs. When our carbohydrate consumption drops, so do our glycogen stores. Several pounds of water are stored along with the glycogen and these are the pounds that are lost when we stop eating carbohydrates. This small amount of weight loss looks great on the scales, but it does not mean much in the long term. Unfortunately, the loss of a few pounds of water does not represent any real loss of body fat.

All nutritionists agree that one of the most important rules of any weight loss or healthy eating plan is to eat *much* more in the way of carbohydrates because they are packed with fibre. High-fibre foods also tend to be low in fat and sugar – another good reason why they are the perfect partner for successful slimming. The bottom line is that we all need fibre. Too little fibre in our daily diet results in the bowels becoming sluggish and constipated. This then leads to further problems such as varicose veins, gallstones and piles. In the longer term, a low-fibre diet increases the risk of colon cancer as the body is unable to eliminate toxins effectively and speedily.

Unfortunately, the average diet has dramatically changed during the last decade. We are eating far more processed foods such as white bread, refined fats and sugars than ever before. We have given up our previous dietary staples, including oats, barley and lentils in favour of low-fibre, convenience foods. By contrast, those living in Mediterranean countries such as Spain and Italy have continued to eat the same foods for thousands of years. The southern Europeans eat many more fresh fruits, vegetables and whole grains in the form of breads and pasta. This has resulted in a much lower incidence of chronic disease, such as heart disease and cancer. Fibre provides the broom to give our insides a thorough sweep and cleans out the colon where some of the most dangerous diseases breed. Eating more fibre is important, not only for long-term weight loss but also for better health, increased vitality and energy levels.

Adding fibre-rich foods to our everyday meals is simple, inexpensive and very easy. Whole grain cereals provide about ten times as much fibre as ordinary Corn Flakes, so a simple switch in your breakfast bowl can dramatically boost your fibre intake. Adding a spoonful of pot barley to soups or eating potatoes with their (scrubbed) skins also makes the most of the natural fibre in cheap, plentiful foods. Eating refined grains such as white flour, however, does not work so well. This is because they have had the outer husk stripped away during food processing. Not only does this remove our fibre, it also leaches away the valuable vitamin E found in the fibrous husk or 'germ' of wheat. Refined white flour contains less than a quarter of the vitamin E found in wholemeal flour and has about a fifth of its magnesium and zinc content. Refined flour is therefore not only a poor source of vitamins and minerals, it is also remarkably low in fibre.

Fibre Facts

Wholemeal bread and whole grains are probably the first things we think of as being high in fibre. But the vitamin-rich fruits and vegetables are also some of our very best sources. Fibre is basically a carbohydrate that is broken down in the intestine and it comes in several different guises. It consists of the cellulose fibres that form the structure of green, leafy vegetables and the outer skins of sweetcorn and beans. There are two types of fibre: soluble fibre, which is soft and spongy, and insoluble fibre, which is coarse and hard. Soluble fibre is essential for successful weight loss as it dissolves in the stomach and helps to fill us up and prevent hunger pangs. Soluble fibre is also important in the upper portion of the gut where it slows down the absorption of nutrients from food. This is no bad thing, as it allows time for vital vitamins to work their way into the bloodstream before the food passes into the colon. Soluble fibre is also vital for regulating the release of glucose into the bloodstream. This means we avoid hunger pangs and sudden sugar cravings as our blood sugars are stabilised. The best way to avoid an attack of the 'munchies' is to make sure we eat plenty of soluble fibre from fruits, vegetables and oats.

By contrast, insoluble fibre has only one main function: to expel waste matter from the body. Insoluble fibre is found in the husks of whole grains, such as brown rice and wholewheat foods. Unlike soluble fibre, this does not dissolve inside the stomach, but passes through the digestive system more or less intact. The role of insoluble fibre is to bind with toxins and waste matter in the system and expel them in faeces. Too little insoluble fibre in our daily diet not only causes constipation, but also means that the poisons the body needs to get rid of daily lurk in our insides for longer. We need to make sure that we eat large amounts of both soluble and insoluble fibre every day of our lives. This will speed weight loss by reducing our appetite. It will also boost our energy levels by speeding the removal of toxins that conspire to make us feel tired and lethargic.

8

Fitness vs Fatness

Regular exercise is the key to renewed energy and vitality. It also gives the body the key to unlock the fat stored in our fat cells. For this to happen, we need to supply the body with oxygen in the form of aerobic exercise. The term aerobic means 'with oxygen' and covers any form of sustained exercise that makes us breathe harder, so we take in deep gulps of oxygen. Aerobic exercise is very easy and does not require any special equipment, expensive gym membership or facilities. Brisk walking is an excellent form of aerobic exercise – provided that it is fast enough to leave you puffing. Running up the stairs is also a good at-home version of the more expensive 'stepper' machines that the good gyms are now equipped with. However, all aerobic exercise must be maintained for a minimum of twenty minutes for the body to benefit. This means that stop/start activities such as golf, cricket and gymnastics do not strictly qualify as aerobic exercise. This is because they do not produce a steady increase in the heart rate that is needed over a twenty-minute period to release fat from cells.

The human body was designed for regular exercise and gentle exertion over long periods of time. It is only in today's sedentary age of the car, computer and washing machine that we are under-utilising our own physical capabilities. Exercise is well worth the effort as it actually increases our energy levels – it won't wear you out, it will make you *more* energetic! Regular exercise increases the enzymes that help the body burn up the fats and sugars in our food. In many cases, the problem of being overweight has less to do with too much fat and more to do with too little active muscle. Improving our muscle tone means we also improve our ability to burn up calories as the mechanics of the body become more efficient.

Developing muscle tissue doesn't make us bigger though. Muscle toning through exercise means your zips will zip up and your buttons fasten without bulging. This is far more important than the reading on your scales. The figures on the scales can be very misleading, for example a lean athlete may actually weigh more that a chubby couch potato. We need to increase muscle weight, not decrease it.

Exercise Calorie Counter

	approx kcal per hour
Step aerobics	600
Skipping	600
Aerobics	550
Swimming	500
Tennis	450
Cycling	400
Badminton	350
Fast walking	300

Stamina Sessions

The benefit of regular exercising is that it increases stamina. This means that you are able to perform physical tasks for longer without feeling the strain. In addition to strength and suppleness, stamina is a useful measurement of our overall fitness and helps determine how quickly we burn up our calories in the form of fuel. Try this simple stamina test each month to monitor your fitness progress. If you are exercising for at least twenty minutes, three times a week, you will find that your stamina levels quickly increase. Keep a record in your diary – and watch your personal fitness levels soar!

Stamina Test

Step 1 Choose a safe, flat route about a mile long (check the distance on a map or with a car milometer).
Step 2 Put on a pair of comfortable walking shoes or trainers.
Step 3 Walking, running (or a combination of the two), see how long it takes you to complete the distance of one mile.
Step 4 Compare your time with the chart below. Keep a note of your time and see how much it improves over the months to come.

Minutes per mile	*Stamina fitness*
20 or more	very unfit
15-20	unfit
12-15	fair
10-12	fit
10 or under	very fit

Finding the Time to Exercise

* The main hurdle to overcome is to START EXERCISING. The only way you will find out how good it feels is to make a start.
* Take one day at a time. Every day try a little more activity. Get off the bus one stop earlier, walk to the newsagents,

take the dog for a run instead of a walk, take the stairs and not the lift. Each one of these simple steps increases your energy capacity and helps burn off excess fat.

* Don't try and do too much in life. If you are too busy to exercise, you are just TOO BUSY!
* Keep a record of your exercising. Make a wall chart in the kitchen or office and fill in the days you exercise, or keep a note in your diary. Try and take some form of vigorous exercise at least three times each week.
* Be persistent with your body – don't ever give up. If you feel too tired to work out one day, set aside time in the evening to go through some simple stretches instead. Make up any lost exercising by doing a little more the following day.
* Be realistic with your exercise goals. Failure is no fun, so be kind to yourself by setting achievable targets.
* Use your time effectively. Look at ways to save time during the day that could be better spent taking some form of exercise.
* Regular exercise is a great destresser as it loosens physical tension in the body and clears the mind. Vigorous exercise also produces brain chemicals that encourage feelings of well-being. Get yourself hooked on that natural high!
* Remember that, in the final analysis, nothing has a higher priority in life than your personal health and well-being. You can only achieve this by regular, vigorous exercise.

The Ages of Exercise

Children

It is important to introduce children to the idea of taking some form of regular exercise while still young. This will help them to maintain a lithe, lean figure and prevent them from developing into lazy, fat adults. Lifestyle routines established now will become the habits of a lifetime. However, it is important not to emphasise the weight-loss advantages to young children. You can score an own goal by making youngsters paranoid about their appearance. Instead of stressing weight loss, highlight the benefits of health and fitness gain. Children will also benefit from improved hand to eye co-ordination and the philosophies of teamwork, co-operation, self-improvement and self-esteem.

Exercise during childhood is doubly important as it stimulates healthy bone development. Fun activities such as obstacle courses, kite flying and games of tag are good for encouraging movement in toddlers and younger children. Older children can be introduced to team games and sports. Teenagers and young children should not do too much weight training to develop their muscles as this can stunt bone growth. Excessive weight training and resistance exercises should be avoided before eighteen to twenty years of age. This is the age when the epiphysial plates seal the tops of our bones with a lattice-work layer to prevent any further growth. Load-bearing exercises can damage the formation of these structures and lead to bone and joint problems in later life. Excessive exercise during puberty can also play havoc with the female menstrual cycle and delay the onset or disrupt periods, and may even stop them altogether (a disorder known in the medical world as amenorrhoea).

Adults

All adults need regular exercise. This is not only important for successful weight loss, but also for better health, stamina and mobility. The best form of exercise is one which leaves you feeling breathless, but that you can sustain for twenty minutes or more. The following are all good forms of aerobic exercise:

* jogging
* brisk walking

* swimming
* aerobic classes
* bouncing on a mini-trampoline
* step exercises in a class or with a video
* roller skating
* team games such as hockey, netball, football etc

Remember that in order for aerobic exercise to release fat from our cells it needs to be sustained for at least twenty minutes, for a minimum of three times each week.

THE ELDERLY

Old age is no obstacle to exercise and there is no reason why we should not continue to be active as we grow older. Many of our bodily functions go into decline over the age of sixty, so we have all the more reason to keep ourselves fit and active. Once we are past the age of 60 our metabolic rate drops so we burn calories less efficiently. Our maximal heart rate reduces as our heart ages, our muscle strength reduces and our bone mineral mass also declines. For these reasons it is important to take it slow and steady when starting any exercise regime.

If it is many years since you took any regular, planned form of exercise, or if you have gained a great deal of weight in recent years, it is going to take a little time before you notice the benefits. However, with time and perseverance you will feel fitter, more mobile and have much more energy. Gradual and gentle exercise are your goals. Non-weight bearing exercises, such as swimming and cycling, are ideal as they involve the minimal energy expenditure. These are a good starting point before graduating on to a more structured exercise routine. Anyone considering starting an exercise programme for the first time in a few years should consult their GP for a medical check-up. This is important as it could reveal factors such as diabetes and osteoporosis which may not otherwise be detected.

Although walking is a weight-bearing activity it is also a good form of exercise. You should always increase your duration of walking before increasing the intensity or pace. Before taking any form of exercise it is well worth completing a gentle warm-up routine. This should include stretches to mobilise the joints and muscles and which will improve mobility and flexibility. Stretching before taking exercise also reduces the risk of injury as it prepares the body for activity by boosting the blood circulation and raising the heart rate for aerobic benefits. For a stretch to be really effective, hold it still for ten to fifteen seconds (without bouncing) before releasing. Always hold onto the back of a stable chair or table to avoid over-balancing. A few simple stretches after completing any form of exercise also reduces the risk of stiff muscles and future injury.

Fluid Replacement

No matter what our age, we all need to drink plenty of water while we exercise. Drinking water to rehydrate the system allows the body to function effectively and enables us to work out harder. Even a couch potato needs to drink around two litres of water a day. This level dramatically increases during hot weather and during exercise. In the hot, humid summer months the body may need as much as ten litres a day to maintain the *status quo*. During periods of intense exercise we sweat up to two litres of water per hour and this fluid needs to be replaced. Drink small amounts of water during exercise and drink it frequently. Avoid drinking caffeine drinks (coffee, tea and cola drinks) shortly before, during, or one hour after exercise as caffeine is a diuretic and encourages water loss. If you feel thirsty your body probably dehydrated twenty minutes ago. Fluid replacement is especially important for pregnant women and the elderly.

12 GOOD REASONS WHY YOU SHOULD EXERCISE:

* Exercise burns off the calories you would otherwise store as fat
* Exercise strengthens and slims the body
* Exercise increases bone density, flexibility and improves posture
* Exercise reduces the risk of heart disease, cancer and back pain
* Exercise helps you to relax, unwind and reduces tension
* Exercise increases everyday energy levels
* Exercise helps to reduce your appetite temporarily
* Exercise boosts your metabolic rate – even when resting
* Exercise improves the appearance of cellulite
* Exercise stimulates the lymphatic system, keeps the skin clear and the immune system strong
* Exercise improves your sex life!
* Exercise slows down the ageing process and keeps you young

9

Family Weight Loss

Children

We can learn a lot about the way our bodies like to be fuelled by watching our own children's eating habits. Kids often find it difficult to finish large meals, but they all love to eat snacks. Nutritionists now believe that snacking throughout the day is OK, provided we are really hungry and not just bored. This shift in our eating pattern is called 'grazing', and so long as we choose low fat, vitamin-rich options, grazing is perfectly fine for a weight-loss regime. The idea is to cut down on monster-sized meals with many courses and aim instead for smaller snacks that will give us a constant energy supply throughout the day. A study at the University of Toronto found that men who ate a staggering seventeen snacks per day were actually in better shape than those who ate three main meals. Not only were these men leaner, but their cholesterol levels were lower and they also released more constant levels of glucose into their bloodstream. In addition, the nibblers reported that they never felt hungry and could give up sweet and salty snacks more easily than their counterparts.

Eating much smaller meals more often helps us to avoid over-eating by keeping our blood sugar levels stable. This means that we don't experience the hunger pangs that make us head straight for the biscuit tin. Eating smaller, more frequent meals works well for children who are used to snacking and it is possible for children to enjoy snacks on good, wholesome food. One way is by dividing large meals into smaller portions. For example, if you usually serve a low fat yoghurt after lunch, save it for snack time. You will not be giving yourself or your child any more calories, but you will even out the energy supply from food and avoid a sudden drop. Fruits and vegetables are not only packed with vitamins, they also make good snack foods. Grapes are ideal for small hands to grasp for example, and carrot and celery sticks are great to crunch on. The occasional refined sugar treat is OK, provided it is just that. Never reward a child with sweets. It is far better to bribe children with exotic fruits, comics, balloons or small toys. This ensures they do not grow up to link sweets and chocolate with good behaviour or associate them with self-esteem.

Of the 140 children's foods launched in 1992, more than half were sugared chocolate, soft drinks and high fat snack foods. In the same year, the food industry spent over £100 million advertising confectionery alone. Sugar companies also fund the Sugar Bureau, which promotes 'education' packs and project material in schools, encouraging the use of sugar in cooking and processed foods. These project packs are fun and highly visual, without a fat person or tooth filling in sight.The highly dubious decision to target children with unhealthy foods is due to the very real 'pester-power' that children exert over their parent's shopping. The National Food Alliance pressure group estimates that 'pester power' is worth at least £1.25 billion a year to the food industry. With two small children myself, I know only too well just how difficult it is *not* to give in to a screaming toddler throwing a tantrum in the supermarket. However hard it is to cut back on the fatty, sugary foods, you owe it to your child's health and well-being to try.

Given the choice, children tend to eat a lot of sugary foods and this is very often at the expense of more nutritious alternatives. The average diet of the under-twelves has been found to be high in fat and sugar and low in vital vitamins and body-building minerals. One study by Professor Rugg-Gunn at Newcastle University found that chips and crisps were the largest source of energy for an average group of eleven-year-olds. Professor Rugg-Gunn also found that their vitamin A and iron levels were low compared to government regulations. In 1990, an additional study revealed that every week the average British eleven-year-old consumed the following: seven bars of chocolate or other sweets, seven biscuits, six cans of soft drinks and four packets of crisps. Few chose to eat any fruit or vegetables at all – so where are their vitamins and body-building minerals coming from?

The food industry will not admit to the damage that these unhealthy foods can cause. Charts produced by SNACMA (the Snack Nut and Crisp Manufacturers' Association) to show the nutrient content of crisps do not even mention the word 'fat'. Their extraordinarily high fat content is misrepresented as 'vegetable' content – presumably because the fat comes from vegetable oils. Lower fat crisps are even labelled with the words 'can help you lose weight only when part of a calorie-controlled diet'. However, as even 'lower fat' crisps contain more fat than chocolate digestive biscuits it would be more accurate to state that they are of no earthly use at all. You can see from these two examples alone how difficult it is to make informed choices about the right foods for successful slimming. When in doubt, read the label to discover a snack's fat content. If this is not listed, contact the manufacturer.

YOUR KIDS NEED HEALTHY EATING HABITS

- Children need nutritious diets to develop and grow
- Life-long eating habits begin in childhood
- Lack of vitamins leads to ill-health in later life
- Tooth decay is one of the commonest childhood ailments
- Obese children have high blood pressure and cholesterol levels
- Good health, vitality and life-long well-being are the best gifts you can give your children

Fat Snacks

SNACK	FAT PER 100G
dry roasted peanuts (average)	49g
KP ready-salted peanuts	39g
Hedgehog lightly sea-salted crisps	39g
Smiths ready-salted crisps	38g
Golden Wonder ready-salted crisps	35g
milk chocolate bar (average)	30g
KP lower fat lightly salted crisps	28g
milk chocolate digestives (average)	20g

TEENAGERS

The British trend for unhealthy eating increases as children get older. The results of a nationwide survey of ten- to fifteen-year-olds commissioned by Channel Four television in 1993 are disturbing. More than 50 percent *never* eat fruit and vegetables, 40 percent eat chips *every day*, and 22 percent of all teenage girls go without breakfast. If over-eating the wrong types of fattening foods is the main problem during childhood, under-eating can be a more common problem in adolescence. Most teenage girls adopt some form of restricted eating regime, whether it is a fad diet, a longer term slimming plan or simply becoming a vegetarian. The problem is that dieting during adolescence can seriously damage health. Any kind of restricted eating inevitable restricts the amount of nutrients available in the diet. Unfortunately, adolescence is one of the key times when we need the best nutrition possible for healthy physical development.

The worry of weight loss is also a common trigger for many serious eating disorders. A survey conducted by the British Psychological Society revealed that girls as young as nine years' old are dieting. Teenage girls are most at risk from frequent dieting and it is important not to underestimate the overwhelming impact of our diet culture on adolescents. As a teenager I was not overweight, yet I counted calories, followed the latest fad diets and agonised over every mouthful. Anorexia nervosa is an emotional disorder characterised by a fear of becoming fat. It has become increasingly common amongst teenage girls (it is rare in males and adult women). Yet we do need some body fat to survive. If a girl's body fat falls below 18 percent of her total weight, her periods will stop and she may even become infertile. Anorexia nervosa involves a total withdrawal from eating, which also dramatically damages the body's metabolism and can ultimately end in death.

One factor in anorexia nervosa is the fear of becoming fat and a preoccupation with food. Bulimia is another serious eating disorder that focuses on an unhealthy obsession with food. The typical binge and purge cycle of bulimics greatly undermines their health, the persistent vomiting rots their teeth and often continues as an obsessive illness throughout their life. Unfortunately, these eating disorders most commonly strike during adolescence at the very time when the body is trying to develop and grow. We now know that most of our calcium deposits are laid down during our teenage years and this is an important factor in creating bone strength. This is especially important for teenage girls, who may become more at risk from osteoporosis (brittle bones) in middle age. Unless we lay down the solid foundations of a healthy body during adolescence, we are unlikely to develop in a healthy way.

The best way to overcome teenage 'puppy fat', regulate weight fluctuations and build the strongest body possible for the future is to adopt the principles of low fat, high vitality eating. Instead of seeing meal times as a battle zone, teenagers can be encouraged to make friends with food and to recognise it as being essential for a fit, strong and attractive body. Learning to cook healthy, vitamin-rich meals is also a top priority. As a nation, we seem to be losing our ability to prepare even the simplest meals. A 1993 MORI poll of seven- to fifteen-year-olds discovered that while 93 percent knew how to play video games, only 38 percent could cook a basic jacket potato in the oven. Asked what dishes they could make, barely half said they could boil an egg and only 67 percent could put together a salad. Regardless of what you like to cook, one of the best moves you can make as a parent is to teach your children healthy, low fat cooking skills that will last them a lifetime.

Adolescence

* Encourage your teenager to cook. Buy an exotic cookery book, delegate cooking the Sunday lunch, keep a scrapbook of magazine recipes – anything to fuel their interest.
* Teenagers eat more savory snacks and takeaway foods such as meat pies, burgers and kebabs than any other population group. Introduce them to the low fat alternatives on pages 65-6.
* Fizzy drinks are bad news for growing bodies as they are high in phosphates which block the absorption of calcium. Teenagers should switch to vitamin-rich fruit juices for the sake of their teeth and bones.
* Watch out for food fads, including crash diets and vegetarianism. There is nothing wrong with healthy, low fat eating or well-balanced vegetarian meals. However, any kind of restricted eating habit needs monitoring to make sure young people get their full share of nutrients for a healthy future.

ADULTS

By the time we reach adulthood most of our eating patterns have been firmly established. We know what foods we like and how we like them cooked. The older we are, the more set in our ways we become. Any attempt to revolutionise adult eating habits overnight is doomed to failure. This *Quick Guide* is about successful slimming *for life*. It does not, therefore, urge you to throw out all the food in your freezer and restock the cupboards with alfalfa sprouts and mung beans. What it does suggest is that you think rationally about the way you choose, prepare, store and cook food for yourself and members of your family. Small differences and gradual changes in eating patterns will make a dramatic difference to both your waistline and well-being.

The Meat-eating Option

These days there is no risk of running low on protein by not eating meat as there are plenty of high-protein alternatives. Good sources of protein include fish, eggs, dairy produce, nuts, seeds, rice and beans. However, meat does contain valuable amounts of iron and this mineral is especially important for women. Iron deficiency is worryingly common in women, especially those who have heavy periods as they lose a significant amount of their iron supplies this way every month. Red meat is by far our best source of absorbable iron and the occasional portion three or four times a month is a good option for the demi-vegetarian. If you do eat meat you should choose it carefully. Free-range and organically reared meat is not only far more humane, it is also better for your health. Animals that are allowed to run free have more lean tissue and less fat than those reared on factory farms. As an example, the fat content of a pig is around 30 percent compared to just 1-2 percent from a free-ranging hog. Factory-farmed animals are also routinely fed antibiotics and synthetic growth hormones and it is the modern unnatural feeding practices that have resulted in the rise of BSE 'mad cow' disease. Although free-range meat costs more it is well worth the extra money. Vegetarian or not, no one needs to eat the amounts of meat that justify barbaric modern farming processes.

Mealtimes

Another factor that features in weight loss is the time of day when we eat our meals. Back in the 1940s, one of the founder members of the healthy-eating revolution, Adele Davis, recommended that we should 'eat like a king at breakfast, a prince at lunchtime and a pauper in the evening'. Her point was that our bodies need refuelling in the morning for the rigours of the day ahead. By lunchtime we need a little more to keep us going, but in the evening we should not overload our digestive systems just before going to bed. Unfortunately, our eating habits are more likely to be the reverse of this, with many of us skipping breakfast, having just a sandwich for lunch and then a large dinner late in the evening.

- Daily calories – burnt as fuel
- Evening calories – stored as fat

The problem with eating a big meal in the evening is that we have no time to use the fuel from our food in the form of energy. If we eat just before going to bed the body shuts down and goes to sleep, stashing away those extra calories in our hips and thighs. This problem is solved by eating earlier and making supper a smaller meal. Try bringing the time supper is served forward by half an hour at a time – just make sure you don't end up eating tea as well as a late night snack! As a last resort, the body finds it easier to convert carbohydrate foods into energy than fatty foods. So if you are planning to eat late one evening, choose starchy foods such as pasta, baked potatoes, beans, rice and pulses which the body will more easily burn off than fats, such as red meat and cheese.

Snack Attack

The snacks we choose have the power to make or break your successful slimming regime. It is so easy to slip into the habit of eating a chocolate bar every day or dipping into the biscuit barrel with every coffee break. The best way to switch over to healthier snacks is to identify exactly *when* you get the urge to reach for something sweet. Mid-morning snack attacks frequently hit us when our blood sugar levels dip. This occurs when we have not eaten enough of the complex carbohydrates for breakfast. Eating a large, vitamin-packed breakfast will curb these artificial hunger pangs and is essential for all those wanting to lose weight.

We often find ourselves reaching for a snack out of habit or boredom. Think of what triggers your motivation. Are you really hungry – or just fed up? It may be that you always have something sweet with a cup of tea or you might always dip into a bag of crisps when you watch a video. The key is to identify these fattening habits so that you can take evasive action. Changing your habits will remove the psychological association with certain foods. The key to successful snacking is to have plenty of healthy options in the house or at work.

Healthy snacks

* Drink herb teas instead of regular tea and replace biscuits with a bunch of grapes or an apple.
* Popcorn is a great low calorie snack, provided you eat it plain without butter, oil or sugar. Keep a bag of

popping corn in the kitchen cupboard ready for when you fancy something crunchy to snack on.

* If you tend to raid the fridge in search of a late night snack, make sure you have a bag of chopped carrot and celery sticks ready for munching.
* If biscuits are your weakness stock the tin with rice cakes instead. They have far fewer calories but make a satisfying snack.
* If you absolutely must have some chocolate, buy a small bar of very dark, plain chocolate which contains less sugar than milk varieties. Limit yourself to one bar a week.
* Seedless white grapes contain plenty of natural fruit sugars and will satisfy the sweetest tooth.
* Alcohol weakens the resolve. If you can't have a glass of wine without a bowl of peanuts, drink mineral water or fruit juice instead.
* The so-called 'diet' chocolate bars and biscuits don't work for weight loss in the long term because they ignore our need to develop a taste for healthier options.
* You are allowed the occasional lapse! After all, to err is human, to forgive is divine. You will have renewed motivation if you learn to love and respect your body.

The Elderly

It is a sad fact of life that as we grow older we tend to grow fatter. Our average Body Mass Index (BMI), a measurement used by health professionals to assess obesity, tends to be higher in the older age groups. This is because we are more likely to eat sweet and fatty foods, such as butter, cream, milk puddings and confectionery. The 1990 *Dietary and Nutritional Survey of British Adults* found that 75 percent of all elderly adults regularly eat biscuits and cakes as against just 30 percent regularly eating pasta and rice.

Osteoporosis

The bone disease known as osteoporosis is a common part of the ageing process that affects about one-third of all women over the age of sixty-five (and some men too). As osteoporosis progresses our bones become thinner and weaker, making them more likely to break or fracture. Eating plenty of calcium and taking regular exercise will help prevent loss of bone mass due to age. This is one reason why this book pays extra attention to both calcium-rich foods and the importance of exercise. Before the menopause, women need approximately 800–1,000mg of calcium a day. After the menopause, women may need as much as 1,200mg of calcium daily.

Dairy products are an obvious source of calcium but they can also be high in saturated fat. The Milk Marketing Board has done such a good job in educating us about our needs for calcium that we often forget that there are many other excellent sources of calcium apart from dairy foods. For example, green leafy vegetables such as broccoli and Swiss chard are good sources of calcium, as are tinned salmon and sardines (eaten with their bones).

In addition to calcium, there is no getting away from the fact that regular exercise is also especially important for mature women. Like muscles, our bones become stronger with use. This is why weight-bearing exercises such as walking or jogging are so useful in later life to strengthen and thicken our bones. A study carried out at Nottingham University showed that regular, daily jumping up and down for the period of a year increased the density of hip bones in premenopausal women by a substantial 3 percent. In this study, the women made fifty jumps a day, which takes no longer than cleaning your teeth. The impact of jumping up and down on the ground seems to be enough to stimulate healthy bone formation.

The side-effect of inactivity in old age is that the elderly find themselves prone to weight gain as they slow down. To compensate for this, more emphasis should be placed on healthier eating. You are never too old to benefit from the many advantages of adopting a healthier eating regime. Indeed, many of the very disorders that affect the elderly, such as cataracts, arthritis and heart disease can be prevented by the unique antioxidant vitamins in food. These include beta-carotene (vitamin A), and vitamins C and E. The British government has finally recognised that more needs to be done to encourage healthy eating amongst the elderly. In 1992, a report by the Committee of Medical Aspects of Food Policy (COMA) entitled *The Nutrition of Elderly People*, made no less than forty-two recommendations for improving eating habits. This was the first in-depth report for more than twenty years and uncovered some disturbing statistics.

The COMA report expressed concern that the elderly were simply not receiving sufficient nutrients in their food to prevent many diseases. It was noted that many elderly people are being admitted to hospital suffering from poor nutrition and that this is not being detected early enough. It was recommended that all elderly people should be advised to eat much more fibre, fruit, vegetables and vitamins A, C and D. They should also dramatically decrease their intake of fat and salt. If the elderly make the simple switch to low fat, high vitality eating, they will not only find that they lose excess pounds, but that they also feel fitter, stronger and are better protected against many of the degenerative and life-threatening diseases.

VITALITY EATING IN OLD AGE

- Take it slowly! Your weight loss will not happen overnight. It may have taken several decades for the pounds to pile on, so they will not disappear in a few weeks. Long-term goals are more achievable.

* Are you too set in your ways when it comes to food? Try new varieties of vegetables and the newer exotic fruits now available. Remember that the more colourful they are, the more vitamins they contain.
* Change your eating habits – if you can't pass a bakery without buying a sticky bun then change your route! If you always buy sweets when you pick up your pension ask someone else to do it for you. If you have always had second helpings, practise saying 'No'.
* If you are cooking meals for just one person, remember that frozen vegetables have good levels of vitamins A, C and E (the ACE vitamins) and are more convenient for single portions.
* Involve your family. If you make the switch to healthier eating let others know so that they won't sabotage your plans by bringing fattening gifts or cooking fat-filled meals.

10

Successful Slimming

Breakfast First

Breakfast is the most important meal of the day for all of us who want to lose weight. The word breakfast literally means 'breaking the fast' and it is vital that we do not to skip this vital part of the day. Having breakfast boosts our blood sugar levels and fuels the body for the day ahead. Nutritional studies in both Britain and the United States show that skipping breakfast is a false economy as our body will under-perform for the rest of the day. This is especially true for children who leave the home with an empty stomach. By mid-morning their behaviour and ability in the classroom is significantly worse than those who have eaten a good breakfast.

So what is the best breakfast? Unfortunately the traditional British fare of fried bread, bacon, sausages and fried eggs is so full of fat that it slides right off the plate and into our hungry fat cells. The very occasional cooked breakfast is fine – but forget the fried bread, make sure the bacon is grilled, poach a single egg and add plenty of grilled tomatoes to reduce the fat content by more than half. Sausages are just too stuffed with fat, rusk, preservatives and leftover bits of gristle to be taken seriously as a form of food – substitute with a lean lamb chop, or better still, a grilled kipper. However, for our day-to-day breakfasts we should be switching to cereals and toast. Not only are these lower in fat, they also contain the important complex carbohydrates that give us a wonderfully steady energy supply for the day ahead.

Breakfast Cereal Chart

measurements in grams per 100g

Cereal	*Total fats*	*Total sugars*	*Kcal*
All-Bran	2.5	19.0	261
Bran Flakes	1.6	18.7	318
Coco Pops	0.9	38.2	384
Oat Bran Flakes	2.4	16.8	357
Corn Flakes	0.5	8.2	360
Crunchy Nut Corn Flakes	3.8	36.3	398
Frosties	0.4	41.9	377
Muesli (average)	5.2	26.2	363
Muesli (no added sugar)	7.4	15.7	366
Porridge (made with water)	1.0	almost nil	49
Porridge (made with full-fat milk)	4.7	4.7	116
Puffed Wheat	1.0	0.3	321
Ready Brek (plain)	6.6	1.7	373
Rice Krispies	0.8	10.6	369
Ricicles	0.5	41.9	381
Shredded Wheat	2.2	0.8	325
Shreddies	1.1	10.2	331
Smacks	1.5	50.0	386
Special K	0.9	17.2	377
Start	1.4	29.1	355
Sugar Puffs	0.6	56.5	324
Weetabix	2.0	5.2	352
Weetos	1.9	33.2	372

CEREAL CHOICE

Many processed cereals are sold with a 'healthy' tag, but just how healthy are they? Surprisingly, some are not as good for us as their makers would have us believe. For example, granola-style mueslis are often high in fat and can contain 45 percent sugar! Even good old All-Bran is 15 percent sugar (and that's before you add an extra spoonful of the white stuff). Kellogg's Special K is promoted as the slimmer's cereal, yet it contains fifty-seven times more sugar than Puffed Wheat. And although some cereals such as Frosties, Coco Pops and Smacks may declare themselves to be 'low in fat' they conveniently fail to mention that they are also very high in sugar (Smacks is a whopping 50 percent sugar!).

Small differences in taste can make a big change to your waistline – Crunchy Nut Corn Flakes have over seven times more fat and almost five times as much sugar as ordinary Corn Flakes. Chosen carefully, cereals can be the very best start to the day. All health food shops offer a good choice of low fat, sugar-free cereals, and supermarkets stock good choices, such as porridge oats, Puffed Wheat, Shredded Wheat and Weetabix. The trick is not to ruin the goodness by adding extra sugar. A bowl of sugar-free cereal with semi-skimmed milk is quick, easy and convenient. It is also a great source of fibre, carbohydrate for fuel and calcium for strong teeth and bones.

THE BIG BREAKFAST

The big breakfast is not to be missed! Choose from the following selection each and every morning:

Bowl of unsweetened cereal with semi-skimmed or skimmed milk *or* mixed dried fruit compôte *or* low sugar muesli with skimmed milk. Top with slices of fresh, seasonal fruit, such as apple, pear or strawberries.

Followed by: one slice of wholemeal bread *or* four low salt crispbreads *or* four low salt rice cakes, spread with 1tsp butter *or* low fat spread *or* 1tsp smooth sugar-free peanut butter.

Served with: one small glass *of* fresh juice, either apple, orange, tomato *or* carrot juice (*or* a combination).

BREAKFAST TIPS

Here are some ideas that the entire family can follow to boost their breakfast each morning:

- Drink an extra glass of fresh juice every morning before breakfast. The best choices are orange, apple, cranberry, carrot and tomato.
- Use fresh bread which is moist enough not to need butter.
- Switch to low fat diet spreads, or use low sugar fruit spreads on bread and toast instead of butter.
- Cereals are a low fat option. Choose sugar-free versions that are also high in fibre (see *Breakfast Cereal Chart* on page 71).
- Add fresh or dried fruit to cereal to boost its vitamin content.
- Switch to skimmed or semi-skimmed milk and save fat grams.

Snacks

Eating a generous breakfast will stabilise blood sugar levels for the morning and means we are less likely to feel hungry. However, regular snackers will find it useful to snack on healthy, low calorie foods during the day to ward off hunger pangs. Each morning, you should choose a glass of fruit or mixed vegetable juice, or a fresh fruit snack. Fresh fruit and fruit juices are the best choices for a mid-morning snack as they are low in calories, rich in energy-giving vitamins and provide a little extra fibre to fill the stomach.

Lunch-box Selection

This section has been included for all those who take a packed-lunch to school or work. Choose from the following list every day:

* 100g (4oz) lean meat, fish, seafood *or* low fat cottage cheese, *or* 1/2 a small avocado
* *with* two thin slices of wholemeal bread, *or* eight crispbreads *or* eight low salt rice cakes, with 2tsp butter *or* low fat spread
* *with* unlimited amounts of tomatoes, spring onions, celery, lettuce, alfalfa sprouts, cucumber, radishes, watercress, carrots and beetroot.

Tea-time Snacks

We all know that feeling we get around tea-time when our stomach tells our brain that it has finished digesting lunch and can't wait until supper before needing some more sustenance. You can be on a diet and still snack – provided it is on healthy vitamin-rich foods. By tea-time we often fancy something sweet and a little bit different. We tend to get sugar cravings at around this time of day as our blood sugar levels begin to dip two to three hours after lunch. This is the time to try a few low salt crackers, plain rice cakes spread with a little Marmite for flavour, or a pot of low fat yoghurt – yoghurts are an excellent choice for slimmers as they are filling and nutritious, without being fattening. Yoghurt is also an excellent source of calcium, a mineral which builds strong bones, and it is especially important for women to maintain high levels of calcium to reduce the risk of osteoporosis in later life. Even in old age, eating plenty of calcium in the diet helps to boost bone density and significantly reduces the risk of stress fractures and curvature of the spine (the dreaded dowager's hump).

When choosing a low fat yoghurt, look at the label to make sure that it contains more fruit than sugar (fruit should come first on the added ingredients panel). Many low fat yoghurts are sweetened with artificial sweeteners and these are fine for those following a weight-loss plan. In some supermarkets you can even find 'very low fat' varieties of yoghurt and these have the lowest fat and calorie content of all. If you want to add your own flavourings, buy a large pot of plain, low fat yoghurt and add unsweetened fruit purées (jars of unsweetened baby food fruit purées are ideal), a scant teaspoonful of maple syrup or a sprinkling of chopped nuts. For those who make their own yoghurts from scratch, use skimmed milk to reduce the fat content and stir in the flavourings once the yoghurt has set.

Supper Time

This is the time of day when it is important to refuel the body after the day's exertions. It is also a time when families are most likely to eat together, or you may be going out to supper with a partner or friends. It is often easiest to focus on eating a carbohydrate meal in the evenings. This means plenty of pasta, rice and starches such as baked potatoes. The trick is not to ladle on the creamy sauces or high fat cheeses. By avoiding meat we also cut down our daily fat intake, often by a substantial amount. Fish and seafood is a good option, provided it is plainly cooked and not dripping in batter – or accompanied by chips! There are more helpful hints on what to choose when eating out on pages 79–82.

The Demon Drink

Alcohol is loaded with calories so needs to be drunk with caution while following a weight-loss plan. Just one pint of beer contains 180 calories, so you can see how easy it is to pile on the pounds by drinking alcohol. Drinking to excess also damages your liver. This is because the liver is like a car with only one gear which always goes at the same rate. Overloading the liver with excessive drinking causes chronic damage as the liver is unable to cope with the extra quantity of alcohol. Although a small amount of 'social' drinking is unlikely to cause the liver too many problems, it will interfere with nutrient absorption. Alcohol depletes vitamin A, the B complex vitamins, vitamin C, magnesium, and zinc. In addition, drinking alcohol also encourages the body to absorb lead and aluminium. While this is not serious in the short term, you should be especially aware of eating vitamin-rich foods while drinking alcohol.

While following your new, healthier eating regime, you are allowed to drink three to four small glasses of wine (or their equivalent) each week. It is best to spread this throughout the week and not drink your allowance in one evening. The Health Education Authority advises that women should drink no more than fourteen units and men no more than twenty-one units, spread over a week – women have a lower allowance than men because of the differing water content in their bodies: in men, between 55 and 65 per cent of the body weight is made up of water, while in women, between 45 and 55 per cent is water. Alcohol is distributed throughout the body fluids, so in men it is more 'diluted' than in women. In addition, a woman's liver is smaller and more likely to suffer damage.

DRINK TO YOUR HEALTH

One problem with drinking alcohol is that it reduces the amount of water within the system. This is because alcohol blocks the action of an antidiuretic hormone, so the more you drink, the more dehydrated you become. The way to drink healthily is to match each alcoholic drink with a large glass of water. This ensures that fluid is put back into the system to replace the water lost by drinking alcohol. Water is especially important for good health and weight loss. Often overlooked, it is important not to forget to drink plenty of water on a daily

Alcoholic Drinks – Calorific Values and Units of Alcohol

	Calories	*Units of alcohol*
Beer, lager and cider		
Half pint (284ml, 10fl oz) of:		
Bitter	90	1
Brown ale	80	1
Strong ale or lager	85	2
Low alcohol lager	60	0.25
Dry cider	95	1
Sweet cider	110	1
Strong cider	100	2
Wine		
Average small glass (113ml, 4fl oz) of:		
Dry white wine	75	1
Rosé	85	1
Sweet white wine	85	1
Champagne	70	1
Fortified wine		
1 pub measure (50ml, 1/3 gill) of:		
Dry sherry or similar	55	1
Medium sherry	60	1
Cream sherry	70	1
Spirits		
1 single measure (25ml, 1/6 gill*) of:		
brandy, whisky, gin, rum or vodka	50	1

* *Northern Ireland and some parts of Scotland serve larger single measures (1/4 gill) which are proportionately higher in calories and count as 1 1/2 units each.*

basis. Water is a natural detoxifier, helping to sluice out the build-up of toxins inside the system by binding them with the fibre from fruits and vegetables.

Drinking water half an hour before a meal also gives you a temporary sense of fullness and helps prevent hunger pangs. The best time to drink water is half an hour before or after a meal. This allows time for food to be efficiently digested by the concentrated acids in the stomach. Try to drink water throughout the day instead of one or two very large glassfuls at one go. Remember – if you feel thirsty, your body probably dehydrated twenty minutes ago. Tap water contains nitrates, chlorine, aluminium and other substances, so it is worth investing in a filter jug, and never use water from the hot tap as it is constantly reheated which affects its mineral content. It helps to keep a large bottle of low sodium (low salt) mineral water on your desk or in the kitchen and aim to finish it every day.

11

How to Survive Eating Out

The basic principles of successful slimming are not easy to apply when eating away from home. Many of our good intentions and much of our resolve can disappear when we're faced with a restaurant menu. It is still possible to follow a diet and enjoy eating out, provided you stick to the low fat, vitamin-rich menu choices. The golden rule is to avoid anything fried, as this will be overloaded with fat – and our fat cells love to feed on fatty foods.

The following guidelines will help you enjoy healthy foods without sacrificing your own permanent weight loss.

British menus

* Ask for a prawn cocktail without the dressing.
* Minestrone and consommé are low fat starters.
* Choose boiled or jacket potatoes instead of roast.
* Skip the gravy, choose mint sauce, mustard or herb seasonings instead.
* Don't eat the skin on roast chicken or duck.
* Request plain vegetables without butter.
* Avoid cooked breakfasts; cereal is a much lower fat option.

American menus

* Choose a restaurant with a self-service salad bar.
* Use mayonnaise, ketchup and relishes sparingly.
* Choose baked potatoes instead of chips and don't add butter or sour cream.

Chinese menus

* Fried rice is very high in fat; choose boiled rice which has almost no fat at all.
* Request boiled noodles instead of fried noodles.
* Tofu (bean curd) is a low fat option found in many oriental dishes.
* Stir-fried vegetables are a good choice.
* Don't be tempted to snack on prawn crackers – they are deep-fried so are high in fat.
* Avoid spring rolls, these also contain a great deal of fat. Cashew nuts are high in saturated fat.
* Beansprouts and water chestnuts are a good option.
* Lychees are an excellent, low fat choice for dessert.

Indian menus

* Curries can be very high in fat; choose vegetable options and avoid dishes like chicken korma which contain cream.
* Indian flat breads are a good choice and better than poppadoms which are deep-fried.
* Basmati rice is an excellent option.
* Avoid deep-fried onion and vegetable bhajis.

Italian menus

* Minestrone soup, melon and trimmed Parma ham are low fat starters.
* Skinless breast of chicken and grilled fish dishes are a good choice.
* Choose simple tomato sauce for pasta and only add a small sprinkling of Parmesan cheese.
* Avoid high fat carbonara sauces.
* Char-grilled vegetables or seafood is a tasty, low fat option.

* Choose sorbet or fresh fruit instead of ice-cream for dessert.
* Cappuccino coffee is high in fat, so an expresso is a better choice.

Japanese menus

* Miso soup with noodles and vegetables is a good choice.
* Soba noodles are made with buckwheat and are low in fat.
* Nori rolls (rice wrapped in seaweed) are deliciously low calorie.
* Boiled rice is usually served instead of high fat fried rice.
* Chicken or beef teriyaki and raw fish sushi are also good, low fat choices.

Middle Eastern menus

* Taboullé salad made with cracked wheat and herbs is a good choice.
* Houmous (made without cream) and yoghurt dips served with pitta breads are also healthy options.
* Vine leaves stuffed with raisin rice, cous-cous dishes and savoury lentils are all good choices.
* Avoid deep-fried falafel and samosas.

Top Tips for Eating Out

* Share a starter.
* Order a starter as a main course.
* Ask to be served a smaller portion.
* Request that any nuts, potato chips, bread and butter or bread sticks are removed from the table.
* Always leave some food on your plate.
* Eat half and take a doggy bag home.
* Order plain vegetables with no added butter.
* Most restaurants will serve fresh fruit or a fruit salad for dessert even if it is not on the menu.
* Mix your wine with fizzy mineral water to make a low calorie spritzer.

Calorie Counter

	Energy Kcal/100g	Sugar g/100g	Total fats g/100g
CEREALS, CAKES AND BISCUITS			
Flour (wholemeal)	310	2.3	2.0
Flour (plain, white)	341	1.7	1.2
Oatmeal	375	1.1	8.7
Rice (white, cooked)	138	1.2	29.6
Rice (brown, cooked)	141	0.5	32.1
Pasta (white, cooked)	104	0.5	25.2
Pasta (wholemeal, cooked)	113	1.3	25.0
Bread (white)	235	1.8	47.9
Bread (brown)	218	1.8	42.9
Bread (wholemeal)	215	2.1	39.7
Biscuits			
Cream crackers	440	trace	16.3
Crispbread (average)	321	3.2	2.1
Digestive (plain)	471	16.4	20.5
Digestive (chocolate)	493	28.5	24.1
Ginger nuts	456	35.8	15.2
Shortbread	498	17.2	26.0
Cakes			
Victoria jam sponge	302	47.7	26.5
Chocolate éclairs	396	26.3	24.0
Doughnuts	336	15.0	15.8
Mince pies	423	31.0	20.7
Scones	362	6.1	14.0
Fruit cake (plain)	354	43.1	12.9
Gingerbread	438	31.8	12.6

Breakfast cereals – see page 71

DAIRY PRODUCTS

	Energy Kcal/100g	Sugar g/100g	Total fats g/100g
Milk (whole)	66	4.8	3.8
Milk (semi-skimmed)	46	5.0	1.8
Milk (skimmed)	33	4.8	0.1
Butter	737	trace	82.0
Cheese (Cheddar)	412	0.1	33.5
Cheese (Brie)	319	trace	23.2
Cream cheese	439	trace	47.4
Cheese (Edam)	333	trace	25.4
Cheese (feta)	250	1.5	18.5
Cottage cheese	98	2.1	4.0
Cottage cheese – low fat	78	3.3	1.4
Clotted cream	586	2.3	59.9
Double cream	449	2.7	48.2
Single cream	198	4.1	21.1
Yoghurt (natural)	79	7.8	3.0
Yoghurt – low fat (natural)	56	7.5	0.8
Eggs (boiled)	147	trace	10.9
Eggs (fried)	199	trace	19.5

	Energy Kcal/100g	Sugar g/100g	Total fats g/100g
FISH (steamed, unless otherwise stated)			
Cod (poached)	82	—	1.1
Haddock	98	—	0.8
Halibut	131	—	4.0
Herring (grilled)	199	—	13.0
Lemon sole	91	—	0.9
Mackerel (grilled)	188	—	11.3
Plaice	93	—	1.9
Salmon	197	—	13.0
Salmon (smoked)	142	—	4.5
Trout	135	—	4.5
Whiting	92	—	0.9
Shellfish (boiled, unless specified)			
Cockles	48	trace	0.3
Crab	127	—	5.2
Lobster	119	—	3.4
Mussels	87	trace	2.0
Prawns	107	—	1.8
Shrimps	73	—	2.4

Note: Fish and seafood contain healthy unsaturated fats.

	Energy Kcal/100g	Sugar g/100g	Total fats g/100g
FRUIT (raw unless otherwise stated)			
Apples (stewed with sugar)	74	7.9	0.1
Apples	47	11.8	0.1
Apricots	31	6.7	0.1
Apricots (dried)	85	43.3	0.6

	Energy Kcal/100g	Sugar g/100g	Total fats g/100g
Avocado	190	1.8	22.2
Bananas	95	16.2	0.3
Blackberries (stewed with sugar)	56	5.5	0.2
Blackcurrants (stewed with sugar)	50	5.6	trace
Cherries	48	11.9	0.1
Dates (dried)	227	63.9	0.2
Figs (dried)	227	52.9	1.6
Gooseberries (stewed with sugar)	16	2.9	0.2
Grapes, white	60	16.1	0.1
Grapefruit	30	5.3	0.1
Lemons	19	3.2	0.3
Melon – cantaloupe	19	4.2	0.1
Melon – honeydew	28	5.0	0.1
Olives (bottled in brine)	103	trace	11.0
Oranges	37	8.5	0.1
Passionfruit	36	6.2	0.4
Peaches	33	9.1	0.1
Pears	40	10.6	0.1
Pineapple	41	11.6	0.2
Plums	36	9.6	0.1
Plums (stewed with sugar)	29	5.2	0.1
Prunes (stewed with sugar)	107	20.4	0.2
Raisins	272	64.4	0.4
Raspberries	25	5.6	0.3
Rhubarb (stewed with sugar)	48	0.9	0.1
Strawberries	27	6.2	0.1
Sultanas	275	64.7	0.1

	Energy Kcal/100g	Sugar g/100g	Total fats g/100g
JAMS AND CONFECTIONERY			
Golden syrup	298	79.0	—
Honey	288	76.4	—
Jam (average)	261	69.0	—
Boiled sweets	327	86.9	trace
Milk chocolate	529	56.5	30.3
Plain chocolate	525	59.5	29.2
Filled chocolates (average)	460	65.8	18.8
Toffees	430	70.1	17.2
MEAT			
Beef			
Average rump steak, grilled	218	—	12.1
Lean rump steak, grilled	168	—	6.0
Average mince, stewed	229	—	15.2
Average sirloin, roasted	284	—	21.1
Lean sirloin, roasted	192	—	9.1
Lamb			
Average chops, grilled	355	—	29.0
Lean chops, grilled	220	—	12.3
Average leg, roasted	266	—	17.9
Lean leg, roasted	191	—	8.1
Average shoulder, roasted	316	—	26.3
Lean shoulder, roasted	196	—	11.2
Average breast, roasted	410	—	34.6
Lean breast, roasted	252	—	16.6

	Energy Kcal/100g	Sugar g/100g	Total fats g/100g
Pork			
Average chops, grilled	258	—	24.2
Lean chops, grilled	133	—	10.7
Average leg, roasted	286	—	19.8
Lean leg, roasted	185	—	6.9
Ham	275	—	5.1
Back bacon, lean rashers fried	332	—	22.3
Back bacon, lean and fat rashers fried	465	—	40.6
Back bacon, lean rashers grilled	292	—	18.9
Back bacon, lean and fat rashers grilled	405	—	33.8
Poultry and game			
Chicken, with skin roasted	216	—	14.0
Chicken, meat only roasted	148	—	5.4
Duck, with skin roasted	339	—	29.0
Duck, meat only roasted	189	—	9.7
Grouse, meat only roasted	173	—	5.3
Partridge, meat only roasted	212	—	7.2
Pheasant, meat only roasted	213	—	9.3
Turkey, with skin roasted	171	—	6.5
Turkey, meat only roasted	140	—	2.7
Rabbit, stewed	179	—	7.7
Venison, roasted	198	—	6.4
Meat products			
Corned beef	217	—	12.1
Luncheon meat	313	trace	26.9
Liver sausage	310	0.8	26.9

	Energy Kcal/100g	Sugar g/100g	Total fats g/100g
Frankfurters	274	trace	25.0
Salami	491	trace	45.2
Pork sausages, grilled	318	1.8	24.6
Beef sausages, grilled	265	2.4	18.0
Beef sausages, fried	269	2.4	18.0
Beefburgers, fried	264	1.4	17.3
Cornish pasty	332	1.2	20.4
Pork pie	376	0.5	27.0
Sausage roll	459	1.2	36.2
Pâté	316	0.3	28.9

NUTS AND SEEDS (natural)

	Energy Kcal/100g	Sugar g/100g	Total fats g/100g
Almonds	612	4.3	53.5
Brazil nuts	682	1.7	61.5
Cashew nuts (roasted and salted)	611	5.6	50.9
Chestnuts	170	7.0	2.7
Hazelnuts	650	4.7	36.0
Coconut	669	3.7	36.0
Peanuts	564	3.1	49.0
Pumpkin seeds	542	1.0	45.9
Sesame seeds	598	0.4	58.0
Sunflower seeds	581	1.7	47.5
Walnuts	688	3.2	51.5

OILS

	Energy Kcal/100g	Sugar g/100g	Total fats g/100g
Corn oil	899	—	99.9
Groundnut (peanut) oil	899	—	99.9

	Energy Kcal/100g	Sugar g/100g	Total fats g/100g
Olive oil	899	—	99.9
Rapeseed oil	899	—	99.9
Safflower oil	899	—	99.9
Sesame oil	881	—	99.7
Sunflower oil	899	—	99.9
Walnut oil	884	—	99.9

Note: Vegetable oils contain healthy unsaturated fats.

PULSES (cooked values)

Aduki beans	123	0.5	0.2
Black eyed beans	116	1.1	0.7
Butter beans	77	1.5	0.3
Kidney beans	100	1.0	0.5
Lentils	105	0.8	0.5
Soya beans	141	2.1	4.2
Split peas	115	0.9	0.3

VEGETABLES (boiled unless otherwise stated)

Asparagus	26	1.1	0.8
Broad beans	81	0.6	0.6
French beans	25	0.8	0.1
Runner beans	18	1.3	0.2
Broccoli	24	1.5	0.8
Brussels sprouts	35	1.6	1.3
White cabbage (raw)	26	3.7	0.2
Carrot (raw)	30	5.4	0.3
Carrot	22	4.2	0.4

	Energy Kcal/100g	Sugar g/100g	Total fats g/100g
Cauliflower (raw)	34	1.5	0.9
Cauliflower	28	0.8	0.9
Celery (raw)	7	1.2	0.2
Celery	8	0.7	0.3
Cucumber (raw)	10	1.8	0.1
Leeks	21	4.6	0.7
Lettuce – average (raw)	14	1.7	1.7
Lettuce – butterhead (raw)	12	1.0	1.2
Lettuce – iceberg (raw)	13	1.9	1.9
Mange-tout	26	2.8	0.1
Marrow	9	1.3	0.2
Mushroom	11	0.2	0.6
Onion (raw)	17	5.2	0.2
Parsnip	66	2.7	1.2
Peas	79	1.8	0.4
Peas (frozen)	69	1.0	0.4
Green peppers	18	2.2	0.5
Red peppers	34	6.7	0.4
Potatoes	72	0.4	0.1
Potatoes (baked)	136	0.6	0.1
Spinach (raw)	25	1.5	0.8
Spinach	19	1.2	0.5
Spring greens	20	0.9	0.7
Swedes	11	3.7	0.1
Sweetcorn	66	1.7	2.4
Sweet potatoes	84	11.6	0.3
Tomatoes (raw)	17	2.8	0.3
Tomatoes (tinned)	16	2.0	0.1
Turnips	12	1.9	0.2
Watercress	22	0.6	1.0

Successful Slimming Progress Chart

The secret to success is slow, steady and sustained weight loss. Don't expect dramatic results overnight – after all, those excess pounds probably took years to pile on. Don't weigh yourself more than once a fortnight and keep this chart to monitor your progress over sixteen weeks (four months).

Starting weight				
Goal weight				
Week 2	lbs lost		total lbs lost	
Week 4	lbs lost		total lbs lost	
Week 6	lbs lost		total lbs lost	
Week 8	lbs lost		total lbs lost	
Week 10	lbs lost		total lbs lost	
Week 12	lbs lost		total lbs lost	
Week 14	lbs lost		total lbs lost	
Week 16	lbs lost		total lbs lost	
Final weight				
Total lbs lost				

Further Reading

If you would like to find out more about low fat, high vitality eating, read *Liz Earle's ACE Plan – Weight Loss for Life.* Packed with tips for life-long healthy eating, the book contains many tasty recipes the whole family will enjoy.

Available from all good bookshops, priced £4.99.

Index